PI

Overcome Negativity Through Positive Energy and
Relieve Depression, Anxiety, Anger, Fear and
Insecurities and Improve Your Social Skills

(Build Mental Toughness and Stop Overthinking)

Elaine Weekes

Published by Kevin Dennis

© Elaine Weekes

All Rights Reserved

Phobia: Overcome Negativity Through Positive Energy and Relieve Depression, Anxiety, Anger, Fear and Insecurities and Improve Your Social Skills (Build Mental Toughness and Stop Overthinking)

ISBN 978-1-989920-82-4

Legal & Disclaimer

The information contained in this book is not designed to replace or take the place of any form of medicine or professional medical advice. The information in this book has been provided for educational and entertainment purposes only.

The information contained in this book has been compiled from sources deemed reliable, and it is accurate to the best of the Author's knowledge; however, the Author cannot guarantee its accuracy and validity and cannot be held liable for any errors or omissions. Changes are periodically made to this book. You must consult your doctor or get professional medical advice before using any of the suggested remedies, techniques, or information in this book.

Upon using the information contained in this book, you agree to hold harmless the Author from and against any damages, costs, and expenses, including any legal fees potentially resulting from the application of any of the information provided by this guide. This disclaimer applies to any damages or injury caused by the use and application, whether directly or indirectly, of any advice or information presented, whether for breach of contract, tort, negligence, personal injury, criminal intent, or under any other cause of action.

You agree to accept all risks of using the information presented inside this book. You need to consult a professional medical practitioner in order to ensure you are both able and healthy enough to participate in this program.

TABLE OF CONTENTS

Introduction

If you are like most people, you probably suffer from vast amounts of stress and anxiety in your daily life whether it's your job, family, money worries or even something mundane like traffic. We've all been there, where we feel furious, struggle to meet deadlines or feel as though we have been unfairly treated. These stressors, big or small, can have serious and far-reaching consequences on our lives, whether it's our health or our dreams.

By utilizing EFT and tapping you will be able to deal with overwhelm, stress and anxiety in a much more effective and efficient way. This will allow you to unshackle yourself from depression, anxiety and even some physical pain, and empower you with positive energy and motivation so that you can live the life you've always dreamed of.

Obviously, it sounds too good to be true, but many scientific papers have validated Emotional Freedom Technique (EFT) and tapping.

It's a holistic therapy that you can do anywhere and at any time by yourself. It allows you to 'tap' into your body's energy and reduce or even remove negative emotions which can have a harmful impact on your health. It combines pressing on meridian (energy) points in the body, positive affirmations and some principles of meditation which combine together in an effective three pronged attack on underlying health issues.

Before I tried it I was also highly skeptical. It all sounded a bit too esoteric. However, circumstances in my life were really bad and I decided 'Why the hell not?'. I jumped in with both feet and was committed to trying it for at least 30 days before casting judgment and to my surprise I found it hugely beneficial and effective. I still practice it

Research by the Centers for Disease Control and Prevention (CDC) estimates that 85 percent of disease is caused by negative emotion. These negative emotions release various stress hormones in our bodies like cortisol that can negatively affect our immune systems; that's why having a positive attitude is crucial to positive health. EFT works by healing the emotional causes that underlie the disease or physical pain.

In today's society too many people are dependent upon pills to cure their illness whether it's depression or anxiety. This can often present more problems through additional side effects and physical dependency. That's one of the great things about EFT, as it is a holistic approach no pills are needed. It can is relatively fast acting and can even make reasonable substitute for psychotherapy which will save you a lot of time and money.

Despite it's rather scientific start, EFT has been streamlined into an easy yet highly effective self-therapy that anyone can use on their own. This book includes pictures, links to videos and step-by-step instructions to help guide you through the routine.

Of course, it's not intended to replace your medical program, but it can be used in combination with it for greater results. I truly hope you enjoy this tapping journey to better health and to a better life.

Chapter 1: Be the Man!

There was once a drunken man who was walking on a quiet street one night. Because of alcohol toxicity, he was totally oblivious of his surroundings; he couldn't hear the people calling him and he couldn't clearly see where he was going. He was swaying like a man who was about to lose his balance. But indifferently, he continued walking. He was nearing home when suddenly he fell off the ground.

Unsure whether it was a cliff or a manhole, he tried to reach out his hands for something to hold on to and successfully grasped a tree branch. Feeling relieved, he cried for help. "Help! Get me out of here!" He was shouting as hard as he could for a minute or so, when a male voice answered him and said, "Let go of the branch. Don't hold onto it." Puzzled, the drunken man answered, "Are you serious? If I do what you say, I'd die!" But the man said, "No. Just trust me. You'll not die."

Afraid of what could happen if he let go of the branch, the man held on to it with all his life. He ignored the pain in his arms and legs and summoned up all his strength to maintain his position. He fell asleep holding on to the branch and was awakened by the rays of the sun shining on his face. Feeling numb and powerless, he looked at the depth below him. To his surprise and frustration, he found out that his feet were hanging 1 foot above the base of the cliff. He then totally let go of the branch and fell hard on the ground, exhausted, and cursing himself.

Many times, people act like the drunken man, who would rather feel hurt than take a risk. When people don't know what is about to come, or what lies ahead of them, they become afraid for themselves. They start playing safe, thinking that it is better to just keep doing what they usually do than take a leap and fail. There are a lot of things people are afraid of, and the story of the drunken man has just illustrated some of them.

Just like the drunken man who was afraid of falling, people are afraid of failures. That is the reason why they don't explore, don't take chances, thus, they don't give themselves the chance of growing up. For many, failure is such a heavy word that they don't want to encounter. When there's one thing that you want to achieve and you fail in the middle of the journey, what do you do?

Some people would stop the journey and go back. Some would stop and stay where they are. But, there are also some people who would continue with the journey. They either go on the same path or take another route. These people who choose to push on are usually the most successful people – the CEO of a top company, the MVP of NBA, or the most inspiring guest speaker in town. Remember that failures are part of being human and they are opportunities for growth and success. When you stumble onto something, don't be ashamed, don't be hopeless and don't stop believing in yourself. Reflect on what happened and learn from it.

Don't be afraid to trust. Just like the drunken man who didn't heed the advice of the man who was telling him to let go of the branch, people usually ignore the most important advices and warnings of all. There are instances when advices of some people seem absurd, but what they don't know is that these absurd advices are sometimes the best for the situation. Imagine that you are driving your car on your way to work and you see a sign on the side of the road saying that you have to take a different route. You ignore it because you know the road well and there is no reason for you to take a detour. Besides, you are running late for work and taking a different route will take much of your time. After a couple of minutes, you find out that a bridge is being constructed and the road is closed for vehicles. And you had no choice but to go back to that sign and follow it. When people ignore the advices given to them, the tendency is for them to make huge mistakes. When fears get to you and you decide to heed them instead, there will come a time when you will regret it. You may not see it in the near future, but that moment will surely come.

When confronted with fears and desperation, don't be like the drunken man who wasted his time and energy holding on to something that he should not have held on to. Instead, be the man who is courageous enough to face his fears. Take a risk and learn from your mistakes. Always stay positive and don't let your fears get the best of you. When you stumble, always stand up, take a deep breath, and tell yourself that you can do better. Take a step forward and another and another and you'll find yourself closer and closer to your goal.

Chapter 2: The First Step Toward Recovery

So you have social anxiety. Now, what? Well, the first step towards wellness is to receive proper treatment. One of your first options should be therapy. Although you may take medications, you should initially try to resolve your problem through therapy programs. Medicines, as you know, can have adverse side effects. We will discuss that later on in this book. For now, let us focus on the types of therapy that you can choose from.

Cognitive Behavioral Therapy

Numerous mental health professionals recommend cognitive behavioral therapy to their patients. Through this approach, people with social anxiety can effectively change the way they think and perceive social situations. It should be noted that the brain tends to adapt to changes. Thus, it is still possible for you to change your thoughts and beliefs even though you have already been used to them for years.

During a cognitive behavioral therapy session, your therapist will expose you to situations that you fear or are anxious of. This technique is known as exposure therapy. It is necessary so you can learn how to react in similar real-life situations. Also, by doing this, you will be used to dealing with such situations. Eventually, you will no longer experience symptoms.

Let us say that you dislike going to the malls, parks, or any public place for fear that strangers might chat you up or give you unwanted attention. Your therapist will let you visualize yourself going to these places and interacting with total strangers. You may even exchange dialogues and pretend to have a conversation. As you become more comfortable talking, you will find your anxiousness lessening.

Your therapist may also practice cognitive restructuring. Through this technique, you will learn how to identify thought and behavior patterns that cause you to be anxious. For instance, you may feel anxious during social gatherings because you think that you are not good enough for the guests even though that is not the reality. You become so engrossed with your thoughts that you are no longer able to enjoy yourself.

Your therapist will help you realize that having such thought patterns prevent you from making a successful interaction with other people. He will help you reassess the way you think and behave when out in public. Once you realized this, you will be able to modify the way you think and act. You will be able to keep yourself from overthinking things. In time, it will be easier for you to mingle during social events.

In addition, your therapist may teach you symptom management skills so you can learn how to handle your symptoms better. Through this technique, you will learn how to relax and calm down each time you find yourself starting to get anxious. It involves breathing exercises that you can do anytime, anywhere. This technique is crucial to keep your mind and body in a positive state.

Supportive Therapy

This type of therapy is typically conducted in groups. So each time you undergo a session, you will be in the company of other people with social anxiety. You will take turns in sharing your problems associated with the disorder. When someone is sharing, it is important for you to keep quiet and listen intently. When it is your turn to share, you should not be hesitant or afraid. Tell them how you think and feel.

Anyway, you can choose between a therapy group and a social support group. A therapy group is more ideal if you have intense symptoms and general support is not enough to make you feel better. During therapy group sessions, the therapist practices cognitive behavioral therapy techniques to help patients address their issues and overcome their social anxiety.

The therapist also introduces methods that patients can use to help them deal with situations that typically trigger symptoms. Visualization, for instance, is commonly used. Your therapist may ask you to visualize yourself in a social event. He may ask you to imagine yourself surrounded by people you do not know. Then, he will ask you how you think and feel about being in that situation.

In the real world, this might trigger your symptoms. However, there is nothing for you to worry about because you are in a safe place. Anyway, as you continue to imagine yourself facing social situations that you are fearful of, you are able to learn ways on how to cope with your anxiety. When you are ready, you can set out in the real world and apply what you have learned through therapy.

During social support group sessions, on the other hand, you will be in the company of people who have anxiety disorders. Since this type of group therapy is more relaxed, you will not be given cognitive behavioral therapy. The group may not even be facilitated by a therapist. Anyone can also be a member even if they have not been diagnosed with social anxiety. They can join as long as they feel that they need support for their anxiety.

What's more, social support groups are not only conducted in person. In fact, you can join social support groups online. The members of the group usually hold meetings on a weekly basis. They also have different schedules to cater to people with hectic schedules or who have a different time zone. You can interact with the other members through chatting.

Hypnotherapy

Hypnotherapy is widely used worldwide to treat a variety of conditions, including anxiety disorders. It is a recognized treatment by the American Medical Association. If you wish to undergo hypnotherapy, see to it that you provide your hypnotherapist with your medical history. You should also have a basic understanding of how it works.

During a hypnotherapy session, your hypnotherapist will put you into a trance. While in this state, you will be highly responsive to his suggestions. Your brain waves start to change and you become more relaxed. Also, your heart rate and blood pressure begin to change.

Your therapist may ask you to recall certain aspects of your life, particularly childhood memories. He will observe how you react to such memories. The way you react can tell so much about your social anxiety. For instance, if you have had a particular anxiety-inducing experience in the past, you may feel anxious each time you encounter a similar experience in the present.

You may even get anxious whenever you encounter something that reminds you of that particular experience. However, through hypnotherapy, you can successfully disassociate yourself from such experiences and see things as they truly are. So the next time you encounter a similar experience, you will no longer associate it with your past experience.

Aromatherapy

Another way to treat social anxiety is through aromatherapy. When you undergo this method, you will use essential oils from flowers, fruits, roots, leaves, and seeds. You can use sedative oils, such as bergamot, cedarwood, chamomile, jasmine, frankincense, orange, mandarin, and sandalwood.

You can also use nervine oils, such as basil, peppermint, and germanium. Furthermore, you can use oils that serve as both sedatives and nervines. These include clary sage, lavender, marjoram, and vetiver. However, see to it that you dilute the essential oils with carrier oils, such as vegetable oils and sweet almond oil.

You can use the essential oils in a variety of ways. You can choose to massage them onto your body or inhale them to calm your senses. If you want to enjoy a relaxing bath, you can add a few drops of essential oil into your bath water. You can also place some on your handkerchief and inhale the scent each time you feel anxious.

CHAPTER 3: How Mindfulness Works?

We are trained to react to external stimuli. If someone comments, you shout back; if the weather is cold, you dislike it; if you're trapped in traffic, you are fuming with anger; and so on. We are controlled by forces external to us. We are never truly in control of our own happiness when we live in reaction to the world around us.

Mindfulness attacks the problem at its root—our habitual reactions to the world around us. As we begin to watch ourselves objectively as if watching someone else, a distance is created between the self and what we perceive. This distancing allows the space and freedom necessary to shape your response - to create our own happiness.

With practice, our conscious response increases and the habitual reaction decreases. Distancing also increases tolerance towards unpleasant thoughts, feelings and situations - we can stay with negativity much longer without reacting. With more practice, the intensity of unpleasantness decreases giving us further control and strength.

If we practice regularly, it will change everything - how we relate to thoughts, feelings and emotions, our attitudes towards life, people, and everything around us. As human beings, it is our right to live a stress-free dignified life away from stress and anxieties - we need only learn to claim it mindfully.

Studies have shown that mindfulness has a positive effect on brain function, lowering the stress response and increasing feelings of relaxation and well-being. It involves being truly present, even during those simple, mundane activities like washing dishes. It can remind you of the "reality of impermanence," Kabat-Zinn writes in his bestselling book "Full Catastrophe Living"[1]. Here you are doing the dishes again. How many times have you done the dishes? How many more times will you do them in your life? What is this activity we call doing the dishes? Who is doing them? Why?"

Practicing Mindfulness

1. Consider what is right with you. Every day, take a moment to thank your eyes for seeing, your liver for functioning,your feet for carrying you from place to place. Heck, thank those mitochondria within your cells for pumping out the energy you need to get you out of bed in the morning.

2. Love yourself unconditionally. Do you hate yourself for being 40 pounds overweight? Rather than setting a weight-loss goal and promising to love yourself once you get there, Kabat-Zinn says you need to make an effort to love yourself "all the way," whether you are 300 pounds or 150. If you decide to eat smaller portions or give up chips for carrot sticks, simply tell yourself, "This is just the way I'm eating now as a way to live better."

3. Live in the present moment. Do not think about what you ate yesterday or make promises to exercise tomorrow. "Every moment gives you the ability to learn, grow, and change," explains Kabat-Zinn. "If you can take a moment and live as if it really mattered, you can take a step back and see those impulses that may be negative to your health.

4. When life gets tough, do not take it personally. When faced with job loss, a foreclosure, or an impending divorce, it is really hard not to place the blame squarely on your own shoulders and get stuck in the "if only" mindset. That sort of rumination sets you up for full-blown depression. While it is important to accept responsibility for your actions, the best way to do that is by looking to the present rather than the past. What are you going to do that is different right now, at this moment, to move forward?

5. Put the "being" back in human. If you fill every moment with frenetic activity-work,

text messaging, household chores, computer games—you never give yourself a chance to simply be. Just sitting for a moment to contemplate the clouds, the smell of freshly brewed coffee, the pattern of stalled cars winding around the freeway, is what separates us from the nut-gathering squirrels. And science shows it's a great stress reliever, to boot.

Chapter 4: The Brain, the Body, and Our Mental State

Until very recently, western science tended to view the brain and body in a "top down" sense, with the higher brain (or neocortex) influencing the lower brain and body, and the lower brain and body having little influence over the neocortex. However, over the last few decades this view has started to change. Now scientists have come to appreciate that the brain and body are constantly communicating with each other and that signals from the body to the brain can have a major impact on all levels of nervous activity. For example, even before you consciously react to a physical threat, such as a rock being thrown at you, your body reacts by shielding itself to cope with the incoming threat. Hence, the way your body and brain unconsciously react to real or perceived threats can have a big influence over your thoughts, feelings, and overall level of nervous stress.

It's also only recently been discovered that the older, more primitive parts of the brain have a big influence over the newer, more advanced parts of the brain. The human brain is divided into three main parts: the primitive brain stem (which we share with many animals, including lizards) the limbic system (which is found in warm-blooded mammals) and the neocortex (the self-conscious part of the brain which deals with abstract thought and is most developed in humans). In turn, this three-part brain system is connected to all the muscles and organs of the body by the central nervous system. Previously, scientists believed that the neocortex has a lot more control over the limbic system and brain stem than vice versa. However, we now know that more nerve signals travel from the limbic system and brain stem to the neocortex than the other way round. This means that it's probably easier to influence our thoughts and feelings via the unconscious limbic system and brain stem (which are more in tune with our body) that it is for us to use the neocortex to calm down our subconscious brain and body.* However, mainstream treatment of anxiety and depression is still based on the dated belief that our moods are primarily controlled by our conscious brain.

*If our moods were determined by the neocortex, then you would expect highly intelligent people to have lower rates of anxiety and depression than less intelligent people. However, studies suggest that people with high IQs are just as vulnerable to anxiety and depression as less intelligent people (and some studies suggest they are actually more susceptible than people of average intelligence).

Chapter 5: Understanding your true nature

Wild animals live on survival mode, they live on instincts, when something attacks them, they run away or fight back. They do not plan about tomorrow or many of the circumstances they meet, they live to survive the day and also to protect their young.

There are times when heavy rains occur or when temperatures get extreme and so animals have no choice but to find shelter or shade just for that period, after the storms, heat or cold is over, they move on with their lives completely forgetting the past tragedies. They are completely at home in their environment

When they are being attacked, their main aim is to survive the moment, if one member of the group is killed, they move on, they do not seek to plot revenge against the killers.

On the contrary, human beings are not like animals. People were blessed with the power of will and the power of thought. People create their environment, they build houses to protect themselves from storms, and they create shelters, swimming pools and air conditioners so that they can deal with the heat.

Human beings plan about their future, they are able to plan and plot revenge if they have too. It is important for you to understand that, unlike wild animals, you have the power to create the life you want.

You have the power to live the life you want, you do not have to live on instincts and accept anything that comes by. You have the power to originate, to exert your will and to plan about you tomorrow.

Chapter 6: What Professionals Can Do

There are a number of ways, which can be used in dealing with stress, anxiety, and depression. We saw, in the last chapter, various techniques used in managing stress, anxiety, and depression. All these techniques can be grouped under the heading of " lifestyle changes". These are means and ways that you can do yourself without much help from a professional such as psychologist or psychoanalyst. However, these may fail to give result in cases of serious symptoms or when the level of your stress, anxiety, and depression is high. There are more effective ways of treating anxiety, depression and stress. These are but conventional methods viz. medication, psychotherapy or combination of these. First, you try with techniques of lifestyle changes. If these do not work or are unable to solve your problem, then you can resort to medication or psychotherapy. Often, a combination of these two methods is used. Using these methods requires consultation with professionals and following their advice and instructions. Medication is a very effective way of managing stress, anxiety and depression including their severe forms. So is psychotherapy. However, combination of these two methods often works best. What follows describes medication and psychotherapy methods.

Medication

Medication is a conventional way of treating anxiety and depression. There are a number of drugs that treat anxiety and depression effectively. All these drugs may be categorized in following four groups.

Selective Serotonin Reuptake Inhibitors (SSRIs). These drugs are used in the treatment of anxiety and depression. SSRIs work by blocking absorption or reuptake of serotonin neurotransmitter by certain nerve cells in the brain. Drugs belonging to

31

this class include citalopram, escitalopram, fluoxetine, paroxetine, and sertraline.

Serotoni-Norepinephrine Reuptake Inhibitors (SNRIs). This class of drugs include venlafaxine and duloxetine. SNRIs work by inhibiting reuptake of two neurotransmitters – serotonin and norepinephine. Thus, these drugs cause to increase the level of these two neurotransmitters, which result ultimately in improving mood. SNRIs are considered as effective as SSRIs.

Benzodiazepines. These are drugs, which are very effective in reducing symptoms of anxiety including muscular tension. Benzodiazepines promote relaxation. Drugs belonging to this class include diazepam, lorazepam, and alprazolam. Benzodiazepines are usually used for short-term management of anxiety. For long-term treatments, higher doses of benzodiazepines may be required.

However, long-term use can lead to risks of tolerance and dependence.

Tricyclic antidepressants. Tricyclic drugs are of older generation and are less commonly prescribed now. These drugs include amitriptyline, imipramine, and nortriptyline. These classes of drugs work by blocking absorption or uptake of serotonin and norepinephrine, which are neurotransmitters. This leads to raising their level, which in turn results in boosting mood. The mechanism of action for most antidepressant drugs is same: changing the level of one or two neurotransmitters in the brain.

Psychotherapy

Psychotherapy is another option of treating anxiety, depression and stress. There are many types of psychotherapy used in the treatment of these mental disorders. These include cognitive therapy, cognitive behavioral therapy, and psychodynamic therapy. Psychotherapy helps the subject in being more aware of his or her own problems: why he feels so and what causes his problem (triggers). Some type of psychotherapy enables the subject to change his negative thoughts into positive ones and change his behavior accordingly. What follows describes some of these therapies.

Cognitive Behavioral Therapy (CBT). This type of psychotherapy is commonly used in the treatment of anxiety and depression. It is based on the concept that our thoughts, feelings and actions are interconnected. CBT focuses on recognizing negative thinking and behavior and changing these positively. Typically, CBT consists of sessions where the therapist helps the subject in recognizing his problems, analyzing these and identifying unhelpful thoughts and their effects. Once identified, the therapist teaches the subject how to change these into useful ones. In other words, CBT consists in learning skills for recognizing and changing negative thoughts, feelings and behavior. The therapist will ask the subject to practice these skills in daily life. CBT finally aims at equipping you with this skill for life so that you use it in daily life. This is how CBT helps you in managing your problems.

Psychodynamic therapy. Psychodynamic therapy focuses on looking into unconscious processes that are manifested in present behavior. This therapy aims at making the subject aware of the influence of the past on present behavior. So, the focus of psychodynamic therapy includes looking into past events that happened especially in your childhood and connecting these with present problem.

Interpersonal and Social Rhythm Therapy (IPSRT). This type of psychotherapy focuses on understanding the working and importance of our circadian rhythm in regulating our moods. It is based on the concept that any disturbances in the circadian rhythm can cause symptoms.

The physician works closely with the subject to understand and appreciate the importance of circadian rhythm and daily routines including eating, sleeping, and working. In IPRST, subjects are taught to track their moods everyday and identify the routines. The therapy focuses on keeping these consistent and addressing any factor that can disturb the rhythm. This often requires building better interpersonal relationships and skills.

Medication and psychotherapy may be effective options of treating and managing stress, anxiety, and depression. However, the solution that these methods provide can be temporary. Besides, medication can have consequences such as dependence and side effects. In the light of these, the best way of managing these mental health concerns lies in the techniques of lifestyle changes or in adopting and following a stress-free diet plan. These methods – lifestyles changes, and diet - can cure stress, anxiety, and depression for life. As such, these are natural methods and do not have any side effects.

Chapter 7: Comparisons and Jealousy

"Comparison is the thief of joy."
Theodore Roosevelt

In this chapter, we will learn that comparing yourself to others can empower negativity and that you are your best comparison.

To start, think of someone, either your friends, your parents, or anyone nearby. Now take this short test:

● Are they better looking for you?
● Are they smarter than you?
● Are they kinder than you?
● Are they funnier than you?
● Are they well-dressed than you?
● Are they more interesting than you?
● Are they more confident than you?
● Are they richer than you?
● Are they more family-oriented and loving than you?

Notice your thinking patterns. You are not alone, many people often compare themselves with others in this manner, some of us may not even be fully aware that we are comparing ourselves at this, or any, extent. It's been around for ages and looking to other people is a natural sense for us to know our personal values of life.

With constant comparisons, we often lower our self-esteem because there is always someone better or that has more than ourselves. We want to be prettier, happier, have more money and things; this makes us feel bad about our own self and causes us to resent and repel others, you start to miss out on great opportunities, friendships, and life lessons. If this sounds like you, you should become aware of when you engage in the act of comparison and jealousy, then act quickly to disarm the negativity. On the contrary, some people also compare themselves to others by seeing everything that they are better at or have more than the next person. This can also be detrimental to ourselves because, as you engage in this act, you are putting yourself above others in a negative way, you are boosting your ego in the short term and it becomes addicting. Happiness, for this type, comes and goes when they have the chance to show off and be better than the next person. This could put someone into a downward spiral of repelling good positive people from their life. You are unique; your gifts and talents are entirely unique to you and your purpose in this world. We are all different from one another and can never be properly compared to anyone else.

How To Curb The Comparisons

"When you are content to be simply yourself and don't compare, or compete, everybody will respect you."

Lao Tzu

Here are some things you can do to learn how to stop comparing yourself to others and feel happier:

You Are Incomparable, Know That.

Why would you compare yourself to others, when you are one out of a billion gazillion? It exactly sounds like a cliché, but the truth is that there's no one else out there who's exactly like you. No one else looks like you thinks like you, or has the same interests as you. You are one of a kind. Comparing yourself to others can suppress your own personal uniqueness and individuality. When you compare yourself to others you are telling yourself: "I should not be myself, I should be more like them." When you're feeling down because you think that you're coming up short of someone else's' life, tell yourself the following:

1. I'm going to become a better version of myself
2. I'm going to start living up to my potential
3. I'm going to become the person I was meant to be.

Life is about being the best you possibly can be, not about being the best in the world and certainly not about trying to be someone you are not.

Love Yourself

Choose to see the imperfections that make you perfect. Own your reality, accept it and be aware of it. These life struggles will help you become a better person, choose to see them as positives and begin the healing process through positivity. You were born with your own set of skills and abilities that are different from others, embrace them, use them, and discover even more, you'll find joy in them.

Be aware of your inner voice, when you catch yourself thinking something negative about yourself, stop, consciously flip it into a positive, do it over and over, it will become natural and the negative thoughts will begin to disappear.

Be Grateful

Next time you're thinking about others and what they have that you may not necessarily have, think about what you already have and how lucky you are to have it.

There are many things to be grateful for and many things to appreciate in life. One reason why we compare ourselves with others is that we are not the person that we want to be. Learning to be grateful is one of the best skills you can have in your life. Instead of thinking of how your best friend has achieved their dreams, think about how happy you are for them. Instead of thinking about how all your coworkers are married and you are not, you should be happy and supportive of them. If you do, you are likely to become good friends and they may be able to introduce you to the love of your life one day. If you are negative towards them, jealous and slowly repel them from your life you may never get that chance. Life is about opening as many doors as possible to see where they take you. Be open to it, think positively and optimistically or you may miss all the chances that you never knew you had.

Compare Yourself with Yourself

Nobody can ever be the best, most successful, most beautiful/handsome person in the world, instead, you should be the best person that YOU can possibly, and there are no limits in life other than the ones we put on ourselves. Instead of comparing your life with others, compare your life only to YOUR life. Think of yourself as the only person you need to impress and prove something to. Have an inner battle with yourself, challenge yourself to be more and do more. Check-in with your own progress from time to time and reward yourself for it. For example, instead of being preoccupied with comparing how much more money you are making than your friends, ask yourself if you are making more money now than you were last year. Instead of being jealous of how successful and perfect your friend's marriage seems, ask yourself if you've made significant strides and improvements in your own marriage and reward yourself and your spouse for them. The more positivity you bring into a relationship the less opportunity you and your spouse have to become angry and make things worse.

Finding Inspiration Amongst Others

Instead of comparing yourself to others in a negative way, turn it the other way and use comparisons as a way for inspiration. Know that you may never be exactly like them and that is not a bad thing, you will simply make your own uniqueness, your own perfect imperfections. Seek out people who are better than you and rejoice that you have these people to challenge you to be a better version of yourself, you can use them as a source of motivation and turn them into inspirations or role models that will fuel your drive to try harder yourself.

Ask yourself such questions as: How can I learn from them? What kind of advice can they offer me? What might I be able to offer them that they don't have?

You must realize that the people you may think are perfect are actually filled with imperfections of their own. Everyone, no matter how rich, how famous, or how many advantages they have. Know that you may not fully know everyone and they may not fully know you, so why judge only using your eyes and ears, when instead you can judge using your heart. Our hearts are always telling us to love one another for who we are, why ignore that?

To sum up, this chapter, try to make progress in your life and look for positive change; be confident in your own life, be grateful for what you have and who you are, compare yourself to yourself, and find inspiration and motivation in others, not jealously. The positive vibes will flow, become addicting and will spread to others. People will respect you for it and look up to you. Cultivate respect both from others as well as your own self-respect, not wealth, power or things.

Chapter 8: TIPS FOR INTROVERTS ON TACKLING DIFFICULT CONVERSATIONS

Do tentative conversation skills get in the way of your work? Does lack of confidence stop you from offering a different opinion, saying no, or asking for what you want? In difficult conversations, does an introverted style keep you from sharing your thoughts in a timely manner?

In "Quiet: The Power of Introverts in a World that Can't Stop Talking," Susan Cain debunks widely held myths about introverts (we're shy, unfriendly hermits) and examines ⏷ualities like reflective thinking and empathetic listening that introverts possess naturally and that are significant conversational competencies.

So why not use your natural abilities and have the conversations you want to have with ease and true connection?

1) Reflect

It helps to think before speaking. Take the time to reflect on your purpose for the conversation. Ask yourself what you want for each person and for the relationship, and keep that in mind during the conversation. Practice in advance with a friend, and take plenty of quiet time for yourself before and after.

2) Ask Questions

Try to ask questions that create an opportunity for the other person to share what's important to them. How would they solve this if they had free reign?

What's the most important outcome for them? Where are their primary concerns?

There is an art to asking honest, open questions. They often begin with: When, Where, How, or What. Notice if there are assumptions embedded in your questions. For example, "What are your thoughts about moving in this direction?" gives the person more leeway than: "Why don't you want to do this?"

The more you inquire about your conversation partner's point of view, the more you'll learn where you have common

49

interests and what a solution might look like.

3) Listen and Acknowledge

Let others speak more than you. As an introvert, you will probably find this to be fairly easy. Just ask a question and listen. It's likely the other person wants to talk much more than you do anyway, so it's a great fit.

Let the other person know you heard them. You could repeat a word or two from the previous sentence, or ask another question: For example, "Can you say more about that?" Or, "It sounds like you've given this a lot of thought."

4) Educate

When you sense your partner is willing to hear from you, think in terms of educating them. Imagine you're living on different planets. They've shown you their landscape. It's tempting to think they should know yours (it's so clear to you, after all), but don't assume. Take the time to explain. For example: "I hear that you think I'm critical at staff meetings, and I can see how it might appear that way. My goal in surfacing potential obstacles is to make sure we create the best product in the most efficient way."

5) Visualize

In your mind's eye, imagine the conversation going well. Play out various scenarios in which, regardless of what happens, you remain confident, calm, and curious. Curiosity is a great ally, and the art of visualization a powerful tool. You are pre-programming your mind for the attributes you want to embody. Over time and with practice, you will become the person you wish to seem.

These tips build on natural traits of the introvert. Use them to be the best conversationalist you can be.

Chapter 9: When Less is More

"If we are not fully ourselves, truly in the present moment, we miss everything."
~Thich Nhat Hanh

What is it that is preventing us from enjoying the "now"? Too many deadlines, too many credits, too many worries - too many fears to handle?

Indeed, to live for today we must think "When Less is More?"

When we focus on doing less and doing it well, instead of doing more and assuming it's better, we're less scattered, and more present. It's not just the goals and the outcomes we visualize; it's the happiness and satisfaction we imagine we'll experience when we get there. So **do less, be more**. Think of what you want to accomplish in life. List your goals. What are you doing at present to honour them? Align your decisions to these intentions and do less of what does not serve you and be more of who you are.

Creating a road map of your life and then making plans to fit them in the little box is of little value. This is a symptom of fear. Often people who try to grasp at plans for happiness tomorrow do so in order to avoid addressing their fears of today. But remember, unless you dissolve the fear it will cling onto you and will block your path to happiness, no matter how much you plan beforehand. Hence **plan less, live more** by letting go of your fears and truly experiencing life in all of its wholeness.

Our "Mafia Mind" or the fear-mind is the real bully. Like a Mafia, our fear-mind extorts joy and potential happiness from our lives by threatening us with what might happen. The past and the future are overrated. 'This' moment is what really rocks. Overcome the fear of unknown (the future) and strip away the past which does not exist anymore. Find yourself in the present and create something beautiful today to 'wow your now' moment. So

dwell less (on the 'what-if' stories), **create more** (space for yourself).

Remember, whatever you pay attention to in your life, increases and intensifies. So do more of what you want in life and less of what life wants from you.

Chapter 10: Tip #3: Before the Exam— Prepare Yourself

Before taking an exam, it is important to prepare yourself not only mentally, but also physically and emotionally to help you perform well and get better results. Some exam takers feel anxious not because they did not study hard, but because their mind, body, and emotions are not well prepared to take the test. Here are some important tips that you need to follow to prepare yourself before an exam.

Learn relaxation techniques

You need to know some effective relaxation techniques that will help you stay calm and confident whenever you feel like anxiety is getting the best of you. You can try deep breathing, by inhaling and exhaling deeply to calm your nerves and to stop your shaking (as well as slow your rapid heartbeat a bit). You can also try relaxing your muscles one at a time to relive the tension that you are feeling.

Another relaxation technique is to close your eyes and imagine things that will calm you down, such as passing the exam with flying colors.

Eat and drink healthy

You should also eat and drink healthy, especially when you are anticipating an exam because a healthy body gives you a clear mind. This is especially important the day before the exam and on the day itself. Your muscles need food and water if you are going to do strenuous physical activities, like exercising or jogging. Your mind also needs the same thing if you are going to use it during an exam. Food and water acts as fuel to your body and brain. While studying, you should drink plenty of water because dehydration makes it difficult for you to concentrate and makes you feel sleepy. You should also avoid drinking soda and juice concentrates that have high sugar levels. Caffeinated drinks, like coffee and energy drinks should be avoided because they can make your anxiety worse.

Get some exercise

It is also important to get enough exercise – the kind that can help you relieve tension and stress. You should make it a habit even when you are not expecting any exam. It is also important to get enough exercise the day before the exam to calm your nerves. You can jog around your neighborhood while listening to upbeat music or you can just let your thoughts wander. You can also listen to audio materials that can help you review for your exam. If you are fit and healthy, you can lower the risk of experiencing anxiety attacks when there is an exam.

Get enough sleep

It is also important to get enough sleep to keep your body and mind relaxed when it is time for the exam. This is why it is important to avoid cramming because it keeps you awake all night before the exam. Aside from that, cramming also puts lot of pressure on you to cover everything that might appear on the exam. Make sure that you get at least 8 hours of sleep the night before the exam. Instead of using the last few hours of the day to review for the exam the next day, the smarter thing to do is just to relax your body and mind, especially if you know that you have already done your best to study.

Change your attitude

This is easier said than done, but it is important to try to change your negative attitude that keeps you from doing well. You should develop positive thinking by visualizing that you can do things successfully. You should also avoid comparing yourself to others because that only makes you even more anxious. What you can do is to write down all the negative thoughts that usually pop up in your head whenever you need to take an exam, and try to cover them up with a positive thought. It is also important to avoid being a perfectionist. Perfectionism only sets you up for disappointment because there is no such thing as a perfect individual. Even the best makes mistakes. Instead of aiming for a perfect score, you should instead give yourself a range like 85 to 100.

On the day of the exam

You should wake up early for the test to give yourself plenty of time to prepare. It is important to have a healthy breakfast that will fuel your mind and body during the exam. Keep your mind focused on the exam and try not to distract yourself by thinking of other things, like watching TV or doing house chores. Make sure that you also wear nice and comfortable clothes that will not distract you from answering the questions. Finally, you should arrive at the test venue early to give you time to settle in your chair and compose yourself before the exam.

Chapter 11: Dealing with Generalized Anxiety Disorder

Generalized anxiety disorder (GAD) is a term used to describe a general abnormality of worrying, irrational nervousness and uncontrollable tension. People with GAD worries about anything that do not even have serious impacts on their lives, from not cooking the dish right to not perfecting an exam. All of these worries come from irrational thoughts of unknown events that all lean towards being negative, hurtful and dangerous.

The anxiety attack of someone with GAD is said to be less than a panic attack, but the symptoms that come with it lasts much longer. Imagine heavy sweating, heavy breathing, dizziness and grumpiness torturing you for almost a day. That is not comforting in any way.

This condition is similar to a phobia, but unlike the latter, the fear is not focused on anything with GAD. A patient can possibly be pessimistic about everything without any basis at all. Soon enough, that person will stop functioning socially.

How will you beat Generalized Anxiety Disorder without undergoing professional treatment and medication?

Mantra

Repeating an encouraging and reassuring mantra is a form of self-hypnosis. It restates your psyche and boosts your confidence to face the world and the future full of optimism.

When you feel worrying again and negative thoughts start to break your spirit, talk yourself out of the situation by repeating a mantra all over and over again. Say something like "Things will be fine because God loves me" or "I've been through this before so I will make it through again" to yourself while practicing a breathing exercise.

You can change mantra depending on the situation. Also, you can try anything that will work best for you.

Mindfulness Meditation

This is a type of meditation where the mind and body finds total peace and unity by mental and physical relaxation. Experts believe that this particular meditation exercise can alleviate the symptoms of Generalized Anxiety Disorder by disrupting the flow of negative thoughts. How does it happen?

Find a quiet place where you can relax, breathe deeply and concentrate in your mind for a few minutes. Keep your back straight and your shoulders relaxed while you inhale and exhale slowly but deeply. Relax your muscles and close your eyes while freeing your mind from any distractions. Just feel and imagine the air coming in through your nose and pass through every last part of your body.

Once you already have physical relaxation and mental stability, start focusing your thoughts on happy memories that elicit positive emotions. It can be a happy out-of-town trip with your family or a scene from a funny movie you watched. It should be anything that will make you feel good.

Doing this for at least 10 minutes will stimulate your brain's prefrontal cortex, the area in your brain that is in-charge in creating joy and peace.

Sensory therapy – It started as a holistic approach in dealing with Generalized Anxiety Disorder but many psychologists have already followed suit and applied this treatment to their patients. Using the senses, you create absolute relaxation and make new memories.

Using your sense of sight, explore new wonderful and beautiful places that can help you in your mental imagery. The aim is to fill your brain with clearer pictures that can elicit serenity.

With your auditory sense, listen to classical and New Age music as studies have concluded that these types of music in particular calm down the mind more effectively. You can listen to any music that you find most relaxing.

With your sense of smell, try aromatherapy by wearing scents such as lavender, rosemary, peppermint and sandalwood. Tasting delicious, comforting foods will also calm you as they stimulate endorphin and anandamide production in your brain.

Lastly, the sense of touch is a powerful tool in beating GAD. Hug whenever you can. Play with a pet dog or cat, or pamper yourself in a bathtub full of bubbles. Getting a massage is also undoubtedly effective.

Chapter 12: Essential Tips for Treating Depression

Before we can look at some ways of treating depression, let us look at some essential tips.

-To prevent the condition from getting out of hand, do not wait for too long before seeking treatment.

-Be physically active; you could also engage in such activities like walking, playing football etc. Such activities make the body to release feel good hormones, which ultimately helps fight the depression symptoms.

-Avoid setting unrealistic goals to prevent stress or depression.

-Try to replace negative thinking with positive thinking to allow your natural treatment method to work effectively.

-If faced with difficult situations where making decisions is hard, you may postpone such events until you are settled then you can make the decision.

-Spend considerable amount of time with people who care about your health, such as friends or relatives, as isolation can make the condition worse.

-If tasked with various responsibilities, just break them into simpler tasks where you can then set priorities based on urgency or your preference. Trying to do difficult tasks and tasks that may seem huge will only make the depression worse.

Natural Treatment for Depression

Nutrition

Omega-3 fatty acids

Depression is associated with lack of omega 3 fatty acids, which are found in walnuts, flaxseed oil, flax seeds, sardines, herring, mackerel, and cold-water fish. These foods are recommended as they boost the level of serotonin in your brain. Other serotonin-enhancing foods include healthy fats such as coconut oil.

Green tea

This herbal remedy contains an active substance known as L-theanine, and works by boosting your mood without any side effects. This active substance has effective properties that allow green tea to cross against the brain barrier. When you drink green tea, it boosts serotonin enhancing transmitters such as dopamine.

L-theanine also inhibits other transmitters such as GABA, a brain inhibitory. To make a healthy drink of green tea, just make a cup of boiling water and add a green tea bag. Allow to steep and then drink.

Intake of B-vitamins

Vitamin B is important in making brain neurotransmitters among them epinephrine, dopamine and serotonin. These neurotransmitters are important in regulating your mood and depression levels. You can obtain vitamin B from turkey, cheese, mackerel, bell peppers, spinach and shellfish.

Magnesium diet

Magnesium is another important part of a diet that is needed to make body enzymes that control different body functions.

Though magnesium plays many roles, the most important function is production of DNA or RNA, and moderation of your heartbeat. Magnesium cannot be naturally synthesized by your body, and has been found to be depleted through stressful situations and depression.

For a magnesium rich diet, try to obtain either a cup of soymilk, a medium banana, about an ounce of dry roasted almonds or cashews and ½ cup of boiled spinach and ½ cup of cooked black beans. The best option is to go for dark leafy greens as well as nuts.

Pumpkin seeds

These seeds contain healthy fats, needed to boost your mood and fight depression. Pumpkin seeds contains L-tryptophan, which is an amino acid required to produce serotonin neurotransmitters. To get this benefit, obtain a cup of roasted pumpkin seeds per day, and sprinkle it by some salt to add taste.

Chamomile tea

You can drink this herbal tea, which is rich in flavonoids. These have relaxing properties. You only need 2 teaspoons of dried chamomile equivalent to a teabag of the herb and a cup of boiling water. Boil the water and add dried chamomile and allow to steep for 5 minutes. If using a teabag, let the mixture steep for 15 minutes. Strain your herbal tea, add some honey or milk and drink 30 minutes to bed.

Avoid coffee

Coffee contains caffeine, which has been found to heighten depression symptoms. Caffeine causes your brain to be exhausted, which in turn disrupts the production of serotonin neurotransmitter, which controls mood. Caffeine actually increases level of serotonin inhibitor 5-HIA, resulting to increased levels of depression.

Other Treatments for Depression
Change your lifestyle

You need to consider why you are depressed, and what changes you can make to your lifestyle to change the situation. Such changes may range from new job approach, better relationship, financial breakthrough or stopping alcohol and substance abuse. Accepting who you are and eliminating those hard-to-achieve dreams can make your life less depressing.

Seek help

Loneliness only makes your life more miserable and stressed up. You should consider seeking help from friends, relatives, church minister, blogs, support groups or a health practitioner. Reaching out to someone you trust can make all the difference in the fighting your depression.

Be positive

Challenging negative thoughts can help in de-stressing your mind through changing how you think. A depressed mind normally leads you to make negative conclusions that are very illogical. When you feel as if no one likes you, ask yourself whether there's any evidence for that. With time, you can learn how to combat those negative thoughts.

Do something new

When depressed, try to do something different, such as going to a museum, reading a book, volunteering for group work or taking a music class. When you change the normal routine, various chemical changes take place in your brain, among them boosting of dopamine. This neurotransmitter controls mood, enjoyment, pleasure or learning.

Have fun

Enjoying what you are doing can lessen the feeling of depression symptoms. Thus, when depressed, make time for things you enjoy. You may plan for things that bring pleasure. For instance, keep going for romantic dinners or for the movies. Be creative in finding ways to keep your mood stimulated, throughout your depression episode.

Exercising

Physical fitness is important in boosting the mood, since it releases important chemicals into the brain known as endorphins. This substance is important in boosting your mood and making you happy. The most effective way of exercising is spending about 20-30 minutes daily on aerobic exercises such as walking, running, or playing ball games.

Meditation

You can adopt a meditation regime starting with 2-3 minutes a day, in a quiet and peaceful area where your mind can relax. Just ensure the area is free from interruptions, by closing the door and switching off the phone. Concentrate on regulating your breathing patterns, and attempt to let go of your thoughts. Meditation is important in boosting your mood and relaxing your disturbed mind, thereby relieving depression.

CHAPTER 14: Conquering Fear and Anxiety with Mindfulness Fear

Fear and anxiety go hand in hand. Have you ever wondered why most little kids are so fearless? They haven't had the time or inclination to create internal stories that make them fear change, rejection, failure, intimacy, embarrassment, abandonment, loss, the unknown, being judged, being alone, losing control, expressing their true feelings, and so many other things that we have mistakenly allowed them to strike fear in our hearts.

Fear is the defense mechanism that we create when we have experienced something that we define as negative. We did not like it and we are going to do whatever we can to ensure that it does not happen again. When we do this, we shut our hearts and minds to all kinds of experiences because, through our fear-tainted glasses, these experiences look kind of like something from our past. We try to control our environment and the people in it in our attempt to avoid the things we fear. Unfortunately, this does not work. There is very little that we can control. This approach also limits our ability to enjoy our amazing lives to the fullest.

As long as we are protecting ourselves from the demons "out there" while changing nothing inside of us, we will always live in fear, regardless of our outside experiences. We will further reinforce the walls that we have built around us.

There are many kinds of fears:

1. Fears we cannot explain like phobias
2. Fears that we keep with us due to past experiences (being rejected, abandoned or hurt)
3. Fears of a future that we wouldn't want (worry)
4. Fears of what others may think of us (fears of success and failure)

Anxiety

Anxiety sufferers do not spend much time in the moment. When the mind is disturbed by high levels of stress and anxiety, it is very hard to focus on where you are, or what you are doing. The anxious mind is always clouded by shadows from past painful experiences or negative predictions about what might go wrong in the future. Anxiety robs us of contentment and of any sense of the present moment.

Absent-mindedness and anxiety are good friends. Anxiety loves you to be diverted and disconnected; it wants you to be scattered, distracted and ungrounded. That is how it works best. Mindfulness and relaxation are also friends. Mindfulness brings awareness of the present moment, it brings roundedness, and it brings a sense of connection and contentment. This state of restful focus is stabilizing and relaxing, and when the mind feels absorbed and relaxed it does not get so anxious.

Anxiety and relaxation are completely opposite states, you will not experience one if you are feeling the other, and that is why mindfulness is the perfect antidote to stress and anxiety. By turning off busy thoughts and engaging in present moment awareness, you can begin to tame and calm an anxious mind and learn to enjoy feeling relaxed.

Worrying and Anxiety

Whether we admit it or not, we all worry. You might worry about the big things, like relationships, your job or your direction in life. Alternatively, it may be small things like your to-do list and stewing over a comment you wish you hadn't made. Worrying is completely normal but when your worries run away with you, it can stop you from really experiencing and enjoying what is happening in the moment. When left for too long, it can also spiral into anxiety or even a panic attack.

Life is fast-paced and you probably find that you spend most of your day in your head, thinking. We analyze, plan and set goals at work, compare, label and judge our experiences and reflect on and evaluate our emotions. Most of us also spend a lot of time dwelling on what happened in the past and anticipating what might happen in the future. The mind is constantly busy telling stories, interpreting our experience by filling in missing pieces of information and then ruminating over the stories it has created, whether or not they are actually true.

When you are lost in worry, it is easy to mistake your fears and worries for facts, instead of recognizing that they are just thoughts. This is compounded when the thoughts become so real that you have an emotional and physical response to them. You may incorrectly attribute a larger meaning to a relatively small action - a friend not calling you back or your boss not saying hello. On the other hand, you get caught up imagining the worst when going for an interview or giving a presentation. Feeling anxious in response to these thoughts can make your stomach tighten; your breathing faster and shallower and your heart begin to pound. Your fingers and toes may feel tingly or numb and you may even feel lightheaded. Before you know it, you are in a full-blown panic, simply in reaction to your thoughts. This pattern can interfere with your sleep, hamper your body's ability to digest and repair, and leave you feeling strung out and exhausted.

We all experience this at times. You are not alone. The good news is that you can do something about it as soon as you notice yourself getting lost in worry, having repetitive thoughts, or feeling sensations of tightness or nervousness in your body. By shifting your attention away from your thoughts and into your actual embodied experience and the sensations of breathing, you can move out of thinking mode and into more of a sensing mode. This automatically alters your physical, psychological and emotional responses.

If you, like most people, also become upset, angry or frustrated with yourself for feeling worried, anxious or panicky, and resist what you are experiencing, you will know that this intensifies the anxiety and only makes it worse. Rather than fight your experience by telling yourself you should not be feeling what you are feeling or trying not to feel or getting upset, it is important to allow yourself to feel however you are feeling. If you can learn to acknowledge what you are feeling and allow it to be as it is for that moment, it is more likely to settle down and pass.

Bringing Mindfulness into Your Fear and Anxiety

There are some really simple ways to start experiencing mindfulness. Perhaps the easiest is to start giving your full attention to the simple tasks you perform throughout the day. For example, you can practice mindfulness while gardening by giving your full attention to what you are doing when planting seeds, digging in the soil, weeding, or watering. You can bring your mind right into the present moment by noticing how your hands are performing the tasks, noticing what you are seeing with fresh and curious eyes, noticing temperatures, textures, and colors. Gardening with awareness is incredibly therapeutic and relaxing to the mind.

Mindful walking

You can practice mindfulness while walking by paying full attention to your feet connecting with the earth, watching yourself move across the ground step by step as you rest your gaze on the path a few feet ahead.

Mindfulness in daily tasks

You can practice mindfulness when swimming, by paying attention to the resistance of your hands against the water, by feeling the temperature, by hearing the splash of your strokes. Notice anything that appeals to you. Be playful, be curious, and let swimming become a truly relaxing and meditative experience too.

You can practice mindfulness when washing the dishes. You can practice mindfulness when reading, just give your full attention word-by-word to an inspiring book or article and be fully and completely present, let the writer speak to you and let everything else wait for a few minutes.

The art of being active and peaceful

Instead of thinking about what you should be doing next, what you should have done before you started, or what you should do next week. You can use present moment awareness to stop it all and give your head a break. You cannot pay the phone bill while you are peeling a potato. So just peel, breathe and peel, breath by breath, inch by inch. Drop your shoulders, relax your jaw and complete your task peacefully. You will do it just as fast, but you will do it without stress.

 By noticing step, by step, every stage of what you're doing; breaking everything down into tiny tasks, you can stop mental overload and anxiety as you involve your mind fully in the day-to-day pleasure of simple activities. Try it, and you will soon feel for yourself what a relief it is to do one peaceful thing at a time.

What to do with negative thoughts

If a thought intervenes, or worry comes to mind, during your mindfulness practice, just try to notice it and let it go. You cannot stop your thoughts, but you can stop getting emotionally entangled in them.

When you listen to your thoughts and engage with them, you start to have feelings about them because your emotions get involved, and that is how anxiety and stress can strike in an instant. When you give your attention to a negative thought your stomach starts churning, your heart starts pounding, and you become disturbed immediately.

The way to deal peacefully with negative thoughts is to notice them, but not get emotionally involved with them. You can practice watching your thoughts in a detached way. Like you might watch people you don't know in a public place. You watch them come and go without any emotional investment on your part. You can do the same with your thoughts. Play with imagining a thought to be like a leaf floating down a stream, see it, and watch it float by, do not get involved, just notice. No energy, no emotion, just watching.

Taming the monkey mind

It is the nature of your mind to hustle from one thought to another. The mind loves to chatter, constantly chewing things over like a puppy with a squeaky toy— especially if you are trying to relax or sleep. But you are not your mind. You know this because you refer to it as "my mind". That means you are the possessor of a mind. And if you own something, you should be able to exert some control over it. If you have a disobedient puppy, you can take it to class and teach it to stop wreaking havoc in your home.

The great news for anxiety sufferers is that you can train your mind. You can learn to be more in control of your thoughts; you can learn to be more peaceful, more grounded, more balanced. You can learn to be more in control of what happens in your own head and stop anxious thoughts in their tracks and mindfulness is a very effective way to start.

Here are three very simple and quick mindfulness techniques you can use to help get you get out of worry, away from anxiety and even halt a panic attack in its tracks.

1. Anchoring

One of the best ways to calm yourself down is to anchor yourself by directing your attention into the lower half of your body. Begin by focusing on your feet and how they feel inside your socks or shoes and against the ground. Expand your attention to include the sensations first in your lower legs and then in your upper legs – do they feel heavy or light? Warm or cool? Tingly or numb? Now include the sensations of your breathing, really relaxing as you breathe out.

This is a great way of anchoring yourself and you can do it anytime, with your eyes open or closed, while sitting or even while walking around. Anchor yourself. Then breathe.

2. Breath counting

This technique can be used in conjunction with anchoring or on its own. Anchor first. On your next in-breath, count up to 6 as you breathe all the way in, and then on the out-breath, count up to 10 as you breathe all the way out. This technique has the effect of lengthening both the in-breath and the out-breath, slowing down your breathing. It also lengthens the out-breath more than the in-breath, forcing you to release more carbon dioxide, slowing your heart rate, calming you down and restoring emotional equilibrium.

Make sure you fit the numbers to your breath and not the other way around. If 6 and 10 do not work for you, find another ratio that does, as long as the out-breath is at least two counts longer than the in-breath. If it is too hard to continue breathing while counting, count for one full breath, then take one normal breath and count the next one.

If you feel very panicked and can't manage the counting, say "in" to yourself as you breathe in, and "out" as you breathe out fully, trying to elongate the out-breath. Then again, say "in" on the in breath etc. Keep going for at least one, minute but go for as long as you need.

3. Finger breathing

Finger breathing is another version of breath counting. Hold one hand in front of you, palm facing towards you. With the index finger of your other hand, trace up the outside length of your thumb while you breathe in, pausing at the top of your thumb and then trace it down the other side while you breathe out. That is one breath. Trace up the side of the next finger while you breathe in, pause at the top, and then trace down the other side of that finger while you breathe out. That is two breaths. Keep going, tracing along each finger as you count each breath. When you get the end of the last finger, come back up that finger and do it in reverse.

This practice gives you something visual to focus on and something kinesthetic to do with your hands as well as focusing on counting and your breathing. It is very useful when there is a lot going around you and it is hard to just close your eyes and focus inwards. It is also a very easy technique to teach teenagers and kids.

These mindfulness techniques are not new. Many psychologists and counselors have been using these tools for years.

What is new is the acknowledgment that we can all benefit from mindfulness—these techniques are useful for not only clinical anxiety or panic but are just as effective for everyday experiences. Try them and notice how much more effectively you are managing your stress, fear and anxiety.

Chapter 15: 30 Minutes to Bid Goodbye
To Stress & Anxiety

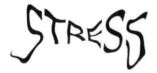

We all experience anxiety at some point in our lives. Stress, as we all know, is good to a certain extent as it helps you to showcase better performance. But, in the present era, all are plagued by chronic stress that deteriorates the quality of life as a whole.

If you feel that anxiety and stress will not affect your physical well-being, then it is time to re-think your approach. Countless studies conducted on the negative impacts of stress prove that it is one of the deadliest enemies mankind is combating. The effects of stress and continuous anxiety leads to various lethal health conditions, including obesity, hypertension, diabetes, fertility issues, cardiovascular conditions, atherosclerosis, and erectile dysfunction, to name a few.

"Yoga has a sly, clever way of short circuiting the mental patterns that cause anxiety,"says Baxter Bell.

It is now time to take action. Make this 20 minute routine a part of your life and you will soon notice the changes...

Warm Up with Breathing Exercises

"When the breath wanders the mind also is unsteady. But when the breath is calmed the mind too will be still, and the yogi achieves long life. Therefore, one should learn to control the breath,"says Hatha Yoga Pradipika.

And, that is why breathing is the key to busting stress and anxiety. The practice outlined below is known as the Breath of Fire. It involves active inhalations and exhalations of equal frequencies with stomach moving in and out with in and out breaths.

How to do:

1. Sit down in a comfortable seated posture, keeping your spine erect and

palms resting on your knees. Allow the tips of the index and thumb fingers to be in contact.

2. Take 5 rounds of deep inhalations and exhalations.

3. Allow your abdominal muscles to relax. Close your eyes.

4. Now start to breathe fast through your nose, keeping the length of the inhalations and exhalations equal. You will feel as if you are sniffing rapidly.

5. Ensure that the breath is naturally shallow.

6. Do 30 strokes at a comfortable speed.

7. Once you complete 30 strokes, pause for 3 rounds of natural breathing and repeat again.

Practice 3 to 5 rounds, pausing for 3 rounds of natural breathing between repetitions. This will take around 5 minutes.

Once you complete the Breath of Fire Pranayama, allow your body to settle down. Make conscious efforts to bring down the pace of your heart beat to its normal rate. Once you are ready, proceed to the sequence of postures.

15 Minute Stress Busting Sequence

1. Marjaryasana - Bitilasana Vinyasa–Cat-Cow Flow

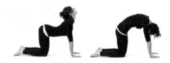

This helps in relaxing the spine and your entire body, thereby plummeting the rising cortisol levels and putting you at ease.

How to do:

1. Come on all your fours, wrists stacked under the shoulders and knees under the hips.

2. Spread your fingers wide, pushing the palms into the mat. Keep the toes extended.

3. Inhale and lift the chin to the ceiling allowing the tummy to move towards the floor, concaving your back.

4. Exhale, round your back, tuck your chin, draw your navel in, and allow the head to face the mat.

5. Repeat 10 times.

2. Balasana—Child's Pose

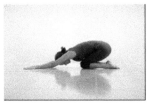

Yoga teachers recommend this pose to calm the wavering mind instantly. It massages your abdomen and circulatory system, promoting better flow of blood and oxygen, thus thwarting your anxiety.
How to do:
1. With the last exhalation in Cat-Cow Vinyasa, sit back on your heels, while folding the body forward, allowing the stomach to rest in between the knees.

2. Stretch the hands to your front and make a pillow by stacking the palms. Rest the forehead on the pillow.

3. Hold the posture, taking long, deep inhalations and exhalations for 10 breaths.

3. Adho Mukha Svanasana–Downward Facing Dog Pose

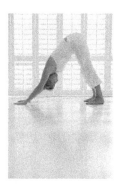

Stretch your body like a puppy and allow your nervous system to cool down with this intense stretching yoga posture. You are free to keep your knees bent, if you have a back or knee issue.

How to do:

1. With the final exhalation in Balasana, separate your hands and stack them under your shoulders.

2. Push your palms firmly into the mat and lift your body off from the heels to come into an inverted V posture.

3. Push your hips to the ceiling and heels to the mat.

4. Adjust the palms to stack your wrists under the shoulders.

5. Engage the core, thigh, and glutes and hold the posture for 5 long and deep breaths.

4.   Malasana–Garland   Pose–Complete Squat

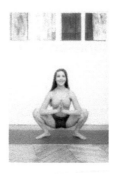

It is a calming pose that corrects your posture and allows the energy to flow through the spine. This, in turn, helps you relax and remain peaceful even during turbulent times.

How to do:

1. With the final exhalation in Downward Facing Dog pose, walk or jump in between the palms and squat down completely.

2. Separate your knees wider than the hips. Lengthen your torso and elongate your spine.

3. Join your hands at heart center, pushing the knees out with your elbows.

4. Close your eyes and hold the posture, breathing deeply for 5 deep breaths.

5.   Paschimottanasana–Seated   Forward Bending Pose

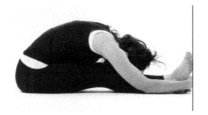

It calms the brain and helps in relieving stress and anxiety by stimulating better circulation to the brain.

How to do:

1. On the final exhalation in the Garland Pose, sit down on the mat and stretch your legs in front of you. Keep your feet flexed towards you.

2. Adjust your sitting bones and elongate the spine.

3. Inhale and sweep your hands over your head and lengthen the torso.

4. Exhale and fold forward from your hips, bringing the hands simultaneously with your body, and hold your feet, lengthening your spine forward. Do not round your back. If you are unable to hold your feet, hold wherever you are

able to reach without rounding the spine.

5. Inhale, lift your chest, and look up. Exhale and fold forward completely, your tummy resting on the thighs and forehead on the shin.

5. Hold the posture for 5 deep breaths.

6. Parivrtta Sukhasana–Simple Seated Twist

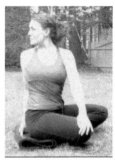

All twists help in detoxification. And, as the levels of toxins start diminishing, your circulation improves and you will become calmer and more peaceful.

How to do:

1. After you complete the fifth round of breathing in Pashimottanasana, inhale and straighten your torso.

2. Sit in cross-legged posture, keeping the spine erect.

3. Inhale and place your right palm on the left knee and allow the fingertips of left palm to rest behind you.

4. Exhale and twist to your right.

5. Suspend your breath and hold the posture, looking over your shoulders for a count of 10.

6. Inhale and come back to the center. Exhale and release the hands.

7. Repeat the same with the other side.

8. Repeat the twists three times.

7. Viparita Karani–Legs Up The Wall Pose

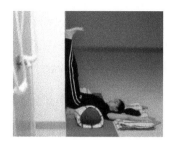

It is a gentler version of Sarvangasana, or the Shoulder Stand. An inversion posture, it is known to help you relax and unwind. How to do:

1. Untwist your torso with the final exhalation and come to the center.

2. Sit against a wall, the left side of your body aligned along the wall. Bend your knees and rest it on your chest.

3. As you exhale, recline on the mat, resting the feet on the wall, keeping the knees bent.

4. Support your body with the elbows. Inhale and as your exhale, relax your lower back and stretch the arms over your head.

5. Hold the posture, breathing deeply, for 10 deep breaths.

6. To come out the pose, rest your knees on your chest and roll to your right and sit upright.

8. Matsyasana–Fish Pose

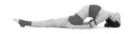

It is practiced as the counter pose to inversions. It stimulates the flow of blood into the endocrine system, stimulating the release of relaxation hormones.

How to do:

1. Recline on the mat, stretching your legs out, and resting the palms under your buttocks.

2. Inhale, lift your head up.

3. As you exhale, rest the crown of the head on the mat, lifting the chest up towards the ceiling. Keep the hips on the mat.

4. Hold the posture for 10 deep breaths.

5. Inhale, lift your head off the mat, look to the front, and place the back of the head on the mat.

9. Supta Baddha Konasana–Reclining Butterfly Pose

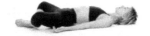

It is a restorative yoga pose that is used for meditation as well. It allows you to restore that natural state of inner calmness and peace.

How to do:

1. After you come out of Matsyasana, bend your knees outward to join the

soles of the feet. You could keep a cushion to support your back.

2. Let your hands rest on either sides of the body, palms facing up.

3. Close your eyes and relax in the posture for 10 deep breaths.

4. Inhale, stretch out the legs and hands. Exhale and roll to your right.

5. Inhale and sit up in a seated posture of your choice and prepare yourself for the meditation.

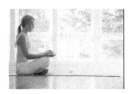

10 Minute Meditation

Studies reveal that spending a few minutes in meditation could help in calming your mind, bringing with it oodles of abundance. It restores your inner peace and calm. You can set your timer for 10 minutes to help you acquaint with the practice.

How to do:

1. Sit down in a comfortable seated poition, keeping your spine elongated. You can rest your back against your wall so that you will not be compromising on your spine.

2. Close your eyes and rest your hands on your knees.

3. Take long inhalations and exhalations and allow your body to calm down.

4. Focus on your breath.

5. Notice how your body moves with each breath.

6. Observe your shoulders, chest, rib cage, and abdomen rising and falling with inhalations and exhalations.

7. Make no conscious efforts to control your breath.

8. If your mind wanders, just return your focus to your breathing.

9. Practice this till your timer goes off.

Once you are able to watch your thoughts and breath without judging, you will be able to calm your mind. Regular practice of these postures, breathing technique, and meditation will surely gift you the potential to stay calm even when the tide is high.

Chapter 16: Zen meditation, How to breathe and sit with the pain

The opposite of the fight or flight response Meditation is one of the most effective ways to combat the acute symptoms of anxiety, period. As I mentioned earlier anxiety is nothing but a prolonged fight or flight response. The body ends up dumping adrenaline and cortisol and as a result you feel stressed. The interesting thing is how effective meditation is at counteracting this feeling.

The reason which I have chosen to teach you Zen meditation is because of its emphasis on posture. I am a firm believer that your body is your mind. This means that not only does your body and your posture change to reflect your mood but by changing your body and learning to have better posture and better breathing you are actually able to change the state of mind you are in. In the words of self-help juggernaut Tony Robbins "Motion creates emotion."

This isn't just some pseudoscience though, modern research has actually shown that there is a physiological basis for why posture and breath are so important in controlling the mood. I won't bore you with the details but when you have good posture it allows you to breathe more fully and by breathing more fully you actually stimulate a nerve (The Vagus nerve) which calms you down. The reason for this is because the Vagus nerve runs through the diaphragm.

How to deep breathe

Most of us think that we know how to deep breathe but the truth is that our bodies are so tense that we are almost unable to breathe deeply. Because of this I highly suggest that you stretch out your secondary respiratory muscles (the ones in the front of your torso) before doing your Zen practice. Here is a short video on how you can stretch your breathing muscles and get far more out of your Zen meditation.

Done? Good, now let's get down to how to actually breathe correctly. You are going to want to sit straight up and down in a firm chair or on a cushion on the ground. Once you are there you are going to breathe so that your body expands from the abdomen up and into the chest. When you exhale you reverse this wave so it feels as if your chest empties of air first followed by the abdomen.

This is the natural way of breathing, if you watch a baby breathing you will see this wave taking place. By breathing in this way you will get more oxygen and massage the vagus nerve. You might notice tingling in your fingers and that is okay, it is just heightened feeling because of the oxygen rich blood.

Posture

"These forms are not the means of obtaining the right state of mind. To take this posture itself is to have the right state of mind. There is no need to obtain some special state of mind."

-Shunryu Suzuki

The way to practice Zen is to do the deep breathing you have just practiced while adopting the correct posture. By changing your posture into the alert, erect posture which Zen encourages you will notice that your mind becomes more alert and clear as well.

In Zen you sit in a lotus posture, the right foot on the left thigh and the left foot on the right thigh. If you can't do this (like me) you can just do half lotus which is placing one of your feet on the other thigh or you can opt to sit in a stiff backed chair instead. The main thing is that you are sturdy.

Here is a short demo:

The next step of Zen is to take your hands and place them in your lap. Place your right hand palm up just below your belly button like a shelf, then lay your left hand in your right with the middle knuckles overlapping. Then touch your thumbs lightly as if you were holding a large egg.

The reason we adopt this hand position is that you will be able to tell if your mind is wandering or if you are putting too much effort into your practice. When your mind wanders, your thumbs tend to mush up like a teepee, when you are focusing too hard and you are stressed your thumbs smash into one another.

The third step of meditating is to imagine that you are being drawn up by the crown of your head (where the top meets the back.) when you do this your chin will tuck slightly and your ears will be directly over your shoulders. This will help you to sit easily and breathe more fully because it will open your chest.

Following this, simply sit and breathe holding the right posture. I know what you are probably thinking by now which is "what do I do when my mind starts to wander?" we will get to that in the next section.

What to do when thoughts pop up

In his book Zen mind beginners mind
Shunryu Suzuki describes thoughts during
meditation as "Mind Waves" he compares
the mind with a pond and how most of the
time our mind is like a pond which is
disturbed by someone and has large
waves. When we sit and meditate if we try
to control our thoughts then it is like we
are trying to smooth the waves by sliding
our had over the water, it just stirs it up
more

So how do you stop thinking if not by
trying? The answer is to wait when
thoughts come, just let them come and go,
watching them and not turning thoughts
into trains of thought. In this way you will
be able to eventually let the pond settle
and be more or less smooth and calm.

This is a great metaphor for how thoughts
work in the brain and it is an attitude we
can carry over into our day to day lives,
when we have negative self-talk, we can

simply sit with it and not pass judgment on the way we are thinking.

So when you meditate, do not try to calm your mind, just sit, watch, and the waves will slowly get smaller and smaller. And when you are anxious, just look at the thoughts that are going on in your head, don't pass judgment, and bit by bit they will go away.

Action item: Practice Zen meditation

Step one: Stretch out

Step two: Breathe deep

Step three: Sit in the correct posture, breathe, and watch thoughts go away.

Step four: Repeat as needed.

Chapter 17:Understanding the Stress Response

Your body has a default biological response to stressors. Some people refer to the stress response as the fight-or-flight response.

When the flight-or-flight response is activated, it has the following physical signs:

-dilated   pupils
-heightened   alertness
-increased   heart   rate
-pale or clammy skin (caused by constricted blood vessels in the skin and sweat   glands)
-less blood flow in the digestive system
-more blood flow in the arm and leg muscles

Let's slow down the process, however, to understand what happens at each step of the response. The stress response process begins when you encounter a threat in the environment. This could be as ordinary as a car cutting you off on the highway or receiving a phone call from a person you are having a conflict with. Your body responds to this threat by activating your hypothalamus, an area at the base of your brain. The hypothalamus sends hormone signals to the adrenal glands which in turn release the hormones called cortisol and adrenaline. At healthy levels, these hormones are helpful for your body. Cortisol increases glucose in your blood to boost brain activity and physical responsiveness. Adrenaline increases blood pressure and speeds up your heart rate which results in a heightened source of energy. Once the threat is over, your body returns to a calmer condition. Heart rate slows down to its normal rate and cortisol and adrenaline levels drop.

The fight-or-flight response also relates to anxiety since those with an anxiety disorder experience a triggering of their stress response when there is no threat or danger present in a given situation.

According to the Depression and Bipolar Support Alliance, people that have anxiety tend to have a more overactive stress response than the average person.

But back to the fight-or-fliught response.

If this process is a good thing, why are we even talking about it? Well, the fight-or-flight response becomes a concern when it is activated for a long period of time. The body's stress response was meant for short-term stresses, to help humans survive and escape difficult scenarios by either fighting or running away. In the 21st century world, due to technology and the high level of comfort Western society has, our biological stress response can be more harmful than helpful in the average person's life.

Long-term exposure to stress hormones like cortisol and adrenaline can disrupt your body's natural functions and they increase your risk for sickness and disease. Some of these negative problems are: depression, heart disease, weight gain, anxiety, sleep problems, poor memory and/or concentration, and digestive problems.

Some additional signs of high cortisol and adrenaline levels are:

-Catching colds easily

-Having a low libido

-Gaining abdominal weight (which can be a sign of too much cortisol)

-Feeling tired, even after getting 8 or more hours of sleep

-Frequent back pain and/or headaches

Chapter 18: Preparing to Meditate

Before starting your meditation, it is important that you look for your meditation space. Find a spot away from all the noise/distractions that may come your way. This doesn't have to be an entire room, it could just be a secluded part of a room. Here are some ideas of where you can be meditating in (this should apply if you are practicing indoor and outdoor meditation techniques).

Find some space in a corner of a room

All you need to have is a meditation chair, a mat and a shoji or pillow to get started.

Find meditation space outdoors

You might find nature's stillness calming and relaxing to help you get into a state of pure consciousness where your body is fully relaxed.

Find a secluded area around the house

If you don't want distractions, you can use the extra room in the house or any other space where people don't frequent to meditate in.

Use a small desk or table to meditate

You will be amazed by how a slight change in the arrangement of your cluttered room could carry you into a new world of meditation bliss.

Optional items to assist with your meditation practice

Once you locate your meditation spot, some like to set it up in a way to help them relax and provide a safe space for meditation. Below are some examples of items you could use to set up your meditation space.

- Candles and incense
- Symbols of peace i.e. talismans
- Items that are meaningful to you i.e. mementos
- Flowers, plants and other living things
- Your favorite music instruments
- Shells and stones that trigger good memories

- Texture, fabrics, light, carpets, chimes fountains etc.

All these should be meant to make you feel relaxed and set you in the mood for your meditation practice. Whatever you have in the meditation space is actually a matter of personal choice, which should be highly dependent on your intuition. Use your heart's desires to have something that is beautiful but that which doesn't distract you from concentrating.

Actually, technology has brought with it numerous tools to help beginners and those who have been doing meditation for years to meditate at their convenience. With this, you really don't even need to set up the meditation space since you just have to visit the online meditation rooms to clear your head up no matter where you are. This can be a quick way of getting rid of all the stress going on in your head.

Chapter 19: Sidestepping A Bad Day Through Distraction

- When life becomes a bit too much to handle and I'm in need of many time out I use a basic technique, that of disruption; and for me at the least, this works a treat. When I do disruption, what I'm really doing is breaking a pattern of my behaviour. What this technique doesn't involve is shopping, telephoning or emailing friends simply because that's what I would generally do throughout my working week. I've listed numerous suggestions beneath that I've used in the past. A number of have been joyful experiences and quite a few worse than the reason why I required a disruption in the first place. As you read each one, write down in order of preference beginning with the suggestion that interests you most (nevertheless remotely), to the last which really should be what interests you the least.

From this list try out the suggestions that interest you the least. Compare how you felt whenever you got out of bed to doing the least favored disruption.

Humor is good, absurd humor (for me) is even greater. Absurd humor works quite well for me and I've usually used it effectively to disturb me from thinking about stuff that have the capability to turn an average day into a truly bad day.

I recall the first time I did a public speaking gig in a huge auditorium filled to capability. Not naturally funny, it was suggested I open my speech with something witty. So I did. What did I hear? Crickets! I responded with "Well moving right along now..."

A few might find experiences such as

this uncomfortable; I found it hugely funny and still do. Moral of this story for me is usually to stop attempting to be funny simply because I'm not - and I think that's hugely funny in itself.

To disturb thoughts that have the potential to produce an unresourceful state, try one of the following suggested disruptions (for men and women) ... greater yet, try all of them if you haven't already:
• Try out a new, intricate and complicated recipe - this will keep you going for awhile particularly if you have to source obscure ingredients.
• Start an embroidery project, one with lots of different colored embroidery cotton.
• Read an autobiography - you might find their 'real' life experiences are much like ours, and occasionally worse!
• Complete a 2,000 piece jigsaw puzzle of water scenes or the night sky.

• Read the white or yellow telephone pages - this will keep you occupied for days on end.

• Choose a little area of garden and count the number of ants, and the species (apparently there are thousands), that run through in a four hour period.

• Count how many tiles you have in the bathroom and kitchen, and then do the same thing backwards.

• Start a knitting project.

• Start a sand art project using either bottles or paper.

• Paint your garden pots - greater still watch paint dry!

• Bake a cake.

• Polish all your shoes and replace all shoe laces.

By distracting your self before plunging fully into an unresourceful state, you might find that good things have the potential to come to pass.

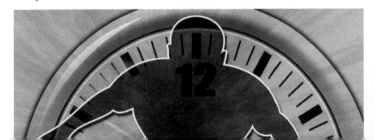

Your knitting or embroidery project could be a winner if entered in competitions, you could invite friends to share your newly baked cake or taste your intricate recipe, perhaps you discover an additional species of ant, and your sand art project could just be the perfect gift for somebody particular.

Chapter 20: Getting to the Root of Stress and Anxiety

Stress might already seem like a normal, everyday thing for you; however, the truth is that you can actually minimize the anxiety in your life in order to stay healthy and be more productive. Before getting acquainted with the different relaxation techniques to keep calm during a straining situation, it is best to understand where all of that pressure is coming from.

One of the main causes of stress is when one experiences major changes within a short period of time. If you are taken out of your comfort zone, you will naturally experience anxiety.

Nowadays, there is constant change, and a lot of people even think that this is a good thing. Yes, change can be beneficial for it paves way to progress but nevertheless it is a main source of everyday stress - whether it is financial, emotional, mental or physical.

Where is the Stress Coming from?

Ask yourself that question and you might already know the answer. Some people worry over how expensive everything is becoming these days, but their paycheck is not keeping up. Others worry about unemployment while the employed feel stressed out over their daily tasks, job security, or annoying co-workers. Work has increasingly become more heavy in this decade as competition is more cut-throat and people get replaced too easily. Moreover, juggling different jobs and maintaining a household at the same time can quickly make someone burned out.

Back in the days, the home used to be a place for rest and relaxation after a hard day's work. However, this is currently not the case for many individuals. Despite technological advancements that make daily chores less time-consuming for us, many changes in the modern family unit have led to a more stressful home environment as well. Both husband and wife are now working and too busy to spend quality time with each other and the kids. Single parents struggle with being the breadwinner and the parent at the same time. All of these lead to disconnected family members and, unfortunately, the rate of divorce is spiking up because of all it. Oftentimes, it is the woman who gets piled up with a lot of physical and emotional stress for having the role of caretaker and earner at the same time. According to a recent survey by Time, over 50 percent of women strongly agree that they tackle more responsibilities at home than their husbands despite the fact that both partners are professionals.

How your Smartphone can be a Culprit

While technology has indeed made lives easier by making things a lot more convenient, it has also contributed newfound stress to our everyday lives. If you look around, people have become more connected with the virtual world than with real life. Sure, we are constantly scrolling down our social networking feeds to constantly get updated, when in turn we are getting more and more disconnected from the actual human being who is right next to us.

Families are quickly becoming more distant as they tend to engage more on their touch screen gadgets than with each other. There is constant stress from trying to keep up with the Joneses as we see regular updates of them online. Technological advancements have opened us up to so many distractions which have actually unplugged us from the real world. All of these build up stress.

Signs that you are Stressed Out

Feeling stressed comes in many levels - from feeling exhausted when you get home to a more serious and deadly heart ailment; the bigger the stress factor, the higher the stress levels, and in effect, the more dangerous the symptoms.

When you are experiencing stress, you feel aches and pains on different parts of your body. Sometimes you tremble and sweat. Oftentimes you experience dry throat. Some experience a stomach disturbance such as constipation, diarrhea, frequent urination or vomiting. You may also overeat or not eat anything at all, develop insomnia, and you may also experience a weakening sex drive.

Emotional and psychological stress dramatically increases as well. One might experience memory lapses, lack of concentration, sadness, impatience, short-temperedness, and constant worry.

Many people turn to alcohol or substance abuse for temporary relief from stress but this will only make matters worse. The psychological, emotional and physical stressors multiply and make your body sick. Your heart and brain can only take so much.

Chapter 21: Use The Power Of Your Emotions

Emotions are the feelings we experience every single day of our life and good emotions is what everyone craves at such a deep level but not many people live in abundant feelings. The majority of the population would rather feel emotions of depression or anxiety and it's not because there is something wrong with them, it's simply because they have become addicted to their problems which cause them to feel that way.

I'm here today to give you a different mindset by looking at all of your emotions in a completely different way so you can start using them when they come up. Part of the journey of life is to feel depression and anxiety by realizing those emotions are there to make your stronger. We need to experience those dark feelings just to make us appreciate ourselves again and feel like we can break out of whatever is holding us back. I never look at anxiety or depression as negative feelings, when I feel those emotions I get to the root cause of why I am feeling that way and then say to myself, 'this emotions is an opportunity to make me stronger.'

If you have been through a dark place in your life or you are currently in a spin of life, then just feel grateful that you are feeling something because most people walk around not wanting to feel again and it's like their a robot. But at least you're letting yourself feel and the distinction I got when I was depressed years ago was, I would never take that experience back because I went through that experience it made me who I am today.

You're not meant to be limited in this world, you're meant to be free every day because the truth is you aren't going to live forever so the time to design your life is now. You can experience everything you want inside your own head it's amazing, I use visualization techniques all the time to attract what I want in my life. If you close your eyes and really focus on all the great things in your life, all the fear will disappear in that moment.

I used to train my mind everyday by visualizing the life I wanted and in a way that felt like I already had it. You don't have to be an expert of visualization to make this work, you just got to feel and see whatever you want every day. Most people do this unconsciously but they focus on what they don't want and you wonder why they keep experiencing it.

Lots of people look at emotions like anger and frustration as negative emotions and tell me they want to stop feeling that way. I love when people tell me they are angry because that emotion is a very powerful feeling to experience especially if you use it to do something productive. Adrenaline is released in your body and you have more energy than you normally do. Most people get angry and just go off at everyone and anything and just sit there frustrated and wait until the adrenaline has gone and their breathing has slowed down. When I get angry I usually go to the gym or I take action on something I have been putting off and with all that energy, you're in a very productive state of mind.

So imagine if you could start turning all of your emotions around and start using them in a positive way. Life becomes easy when you start being in control of your emotions and having fun with them.

I used to be friends with someone who was so angry all the time that he couldn't cope with anything; he would just lose it at everyone and anything. I was happy he was letting his anger out because most people repress this emotion and this is what causes depression because you feel depressed when you repress anger. The fact that he was letting himself go there I was happy and I showed him some techniques to help him harness the emotion and direct it into bettering himself.

He has completely transformed his life around just because he is now conscious of the emotions he feels and he uses them when they come up. All that took was him not repressing his emotions anymore and really feeling what's coming up and figuring out an action to take. Most people that lift weights have told me that they try to psych themselves up before going in for a lift. Natural adrenaline shoots through their body so they get the best out of themselves.

So this first chapter is all about getting inside your head whatever emotions you have been going through lately it's time to look at them in a different way and use what you know now to harness them for good. I'm going to give you a visualisation technique so you can use this every morning to feel whatever emotions you want so you can attract the life of your dreams.

Feel Rich Now Technique

1. Make a list of all the emotional states that you believe feeling rich would give you? Example: Freedom, Confidence, Happiness etc.

2. Choose the first state on your list. Remember a time when you really felt that way. Fully return to it now- see what you saw, hear what you heard and feel how you felt. Keep going through this memory, make the colours brighter and richer, the sounds louder and feeling stronger

3. As you feel these feelings, squeeze your thumb and middle finger together and say 'I am Rich!' In Your mind or out loud.

4. Repeat steps 2-3 with each emotional state on your list. Soon just squeezing your thumb and middle finger together and repeating the phrase 'I am Rich!' Will begin to bring back all those good feelings with associate to being rich.

This is your anchor that you will use when you want to feel rich at any time.

If you can get good control over your emotions and start enjoying them when they come up there is absolutely nothing you can't do. Mastering your emotions is a skillset and it takes as much work as staying healthy but it gets easier as you progress. Sometime your emotions will hold you back if you let them but they can also be turned around very easily. It's all about you stopping the story that you aren't in control and start moving towards a life that you want to live and it starts with you.

You don't have to live in social fear anymore if you make a decision right now to change. You could start being your charismatic self and start changing who you are. One of the things that I live for in this life is seeing someone that has a social phobia and seeing them a year or two later completely transformed. They look you in the eye, they talk with confidence and it inspires me to better myself. Your life can change drastically in a years' time if you take advantage and realize you're in control. Become the person now that others will remember you for later.

Chapter 22: Yoga

Yoga originated from India. It is a physical, mental and spiritual practice which is not religious but usually associated with Buddhism and Hinduism. It can also be associated with meditation, because of its breathing exercises combined with yoga poses. It is popular because of its health benefits, not just for distressing, but also for losing weight. It is a great relaxation technique to relieve from stress, because it conditions the mental and the physical estate of the body.

Yoga has many branches and lineages, but the most popular and practiced nowadays is the "flow yoga," where yoga poses are performed within a slow pace accompanied with regulated breathing. The breathing exercises combined with the yoga poses help the mind and body renew their health and therefore give a feeling of ease. It is important that breathing through the nose is practiced during yoga. Practitioners believe that breathing through the nose filters the air that comes into the lungs while making it moist and warm. It is said that with this technique, the flow of vital energy in the body is promoted, therefore relieving stress.

Yoga poses or asanas tone up the entire system, not just the body but also the mind. They provide internal massage and pressure to the internal organs such as the liver, stomach and lungs by improving the blood circulation all through these organs. This keeps all the organs healthy and with its best operating condition.

For example, the shoulder stand, where the feet are raised to the sky while the body is supported by the shoulder, relieves tension on abdominal organs and muscles. It also allows clogged pelvic and leg veins drain down as if draining down the tension and stress from the leg muscles. People who do yoga say they changed their perspective into a more positive outlook in life by feeling better about themselves. It also helps them keep calm even in strenuous situations.

Chapter 23: HEADACHES AND MIGRAINES

Headaches, also known as Cephalalgia, are defined as the pain felt in any area of the head or neck. The presence of pain can last for some time and can even extend to the neck. Records show that 90% of the human populace is likely to suffer from headaches during any given year. Of this number, 1% is reported to experience serious headache conditions. While headaches may seem like a simple pain that is curable using over-the-counter medicines, this condition requires attention, especially if experienced regularly. Migraines, on the other hand, are classified as a throbbing pain in the head which exhibits pulsating and recurring sensations. With its almost similar characteristics, the migraine and common headache often overlap. To provide distinction, it is important to look at the intensity of pain felt in both conditions.

Tension headaches, the most common type of headaches, result in a dull or squeezing pressing pain in the head. The sensation can be similar to putting an extremely tight band around the head. It usually starts at the back of the head and gradually spreads forward. The pain is just mild to moderate and not altogether disabling. A person can still function normally with a tension headache. The pain is tolerable and can happen anytime. Tension headaches can even occur daily to some people.

Migraines involve extreme throbbing, pulsating, or pounding pain in the head that is often accompanied by nausea, vomiting, and increased sensitivity to light (Photophobia) and sound (Phonophobia). Simply put, the gravity of pain in a migraine is more intense and severe than that of a tension headache. In terms of location of pain, a tension headache is more generalized, encompassing most areas such as the scalp, forehead, back of

143

the neck, and temples; the pain is located on both sides of the head, whereas, a migraine affects only one side of the head and usually focuses near the eye closest to the affected area. Migraines are sometimes preceded by warning symptoms, called aura, which include blind spots, light flashes, and a tingling of the extremities.

A tension headache usually occurs as a symptom of an existing condition that involves the head and the neck. The presence of pain is attributed to the disruption in the structures around the brain. Technically, the pain is caused by the irritation and disruption of several nerve endings which may result in the inflammation of blood vessels around the surface of the brain. There are nine pain-sensitive areas in the brain that make a person susceptible to headaches. These are the skull, mucous membranes, ears, muscles, arteries, nerves, subcutaneous tissues, sinuses, and eyes. According to the

International Classification of Headache Disorders, there are 13 official classifications of headaches. The first 4 classifications fall under Primary Headache, the next 7 are known as Secondary Headaches, and the last two groups are further divided into two more sub-classifications which are Primary Facial Pain and Other Headaches. Of these classifications, the Primary Headache is the most rampant. Tension headaches and migraines fall under this category.

As previously stressed, a headache can be a symptom of an existing health problem. It can also be the side-effect of taking a prescribed medication. It is important to note that a headache can be induced by many factors. Most of these relate to psychological, biological, and environmental factors. Some of the most known causes of headaches are persistent stress, tension, depression, or anxiety. Various psychological factors like over fatigue and anxiety may further contribute to the development of a headache. Daily activities that trigger mechanical problems in the body such as neck strain can also induce pain in the head. People suffering from a sinus infection may also experience a period of headaches that usually occurs during the body's attempt to fight the sinus infection. In addition, hormonal factors can further lead to a headache. Women are more prone to tension headaches and migraines than men. Studies have shown that there is a link between migraines and hormonal fluctuations experienced by women during their menstrual cycle. Women in their menopausal years usually do not experience migraines any longer. Studies also suggest that some components in processed food and drinks containing Tyramine can induce a tension headache. In serious cases, a headache can be a symptom of diseases or conditions involving the central nervous system. Brain tumors, hemorrhage, or CNS infections may also trigger pain the head.

Like headaches, migraines can also be triggered by different underlying factors. The genetics of an individual give a 51% likelihood of determining whether he or she will suffer from migraines. Life events related to psychological factors, such as the menopausal period or a pregnancy, may further trigger migraines. Aside from this, using oral contraceptives and other related drugs may include a migraine as one of the side effects.

While headaches and migraines are commonly managed using self-medication, patients are recommended to consult a doctor especially in cases of prolonged and extreme pain. Secondary headaches are headaches caused by other underlying conditions such as high blood pressure, head injury, tumor, or infections like meningitis or encephalitis. This type of headache needs serious diagnostic approaches. Doctors may require their patients to keep a "headache diary" to help them determine the type of headache he or she is experiencing and its underlying causes. Blood tests may also be performed. Computerized Tomography (CT scan) or Magnetic Resonance Imaging (MRI) may also be taken in order to properly view the structures of the brain especially for signs of a tumor, an aneurysm, a blood clot, or bleeding. Evidence of a previous stroke can also be detected using these methods. Brain scans are also advised for people aged 50 and above because headaches experienced by older people can be a sign of a tumor or a stroke. If the headache or migraine is suspected to be caused by an existing condition, doctors may also perform a Spinal Tap or a Lumbar Puncture. Under these procedures, a needle is inserted in between the vertebrae at the lumbar area or lower back to extricate a test of cerebrospinal fluid (CSF). Examining the fluid can also determine if there is the presence of an infection such as meningitis.

There are many treatments for headaches and migraines among which are over-the-counter medicines. People suffering from mild headaches often resort to these treatments because of its cost-efficiency and convenience. The most common over-the-counter drugs to treat tension headaches include aspirin, ibuprofen (Motrin, Advil), acetaminophen (Tylenol), and naproxen (Aleve). However, severe conditions may require a doctor's prescription. Some of these medications include meperidine (Demerol), codeine, triptans, ergot derivatives, dopamine antagonists, and serotonin agonists among others. It is important to remember that some medications may narrow blood vessels to treat a migraine headache. If you have heart disease, this medication is dangerous for you. Other drugs can also be dangerous if taken during pregnancy;

thus, you need to consult your doctor first before you start taking these drugs.

For cheaper and alternative headache treatments, experts suggest some possible home remedies. These treatments, which are usually found in the kitchen, include fish oil, peppermint oil, caffeine, and ginger (or ginger capsules). One may also consider getting a nice head massage to alleviate the pain. If the pain is due to stress, one may consider getting enough bed rest to restore the body's functions. A change in lifestyle can be another way to manage headaches such as getting enough sleep (7-8 hours a day), avoiding strenuous jobs, drinking a lot of water, avoid drinking too much alcohol, and not smoking. Oftentimes, psychological factors trigger the pain; thus, it is recommended to encourage stress-free thoughts and engage in stimulating thinking sessions instead. Spend time to unwind with friends to avoid stress. Give yourself a break once in a while.

Chapter 24: Self-help Techniques

There are also a number of self-help techniques that for a person can try on their own time. These have been known to work on certain people since they are completely person-oriented. But these techniques are definitely worth a try!

Consider the affect on your life

Perhaps some of these memories will be painful for you to look back on, but they are definitely worth it if you can get the strength you need from them. Think back on some unhappy memories that you may have because you were afraid to face your uncertainties, some opportunities that you missed, some moments that you can never get back.

Did you ever stop yourself from asking out a girl you liked because you were scared of rejection? Did you stop from pitching a plan at your monthly office meeting because you were afraid of being laughed at? Did you not audition for the role of

Juliet at high school before you were afraid of being on stage even though you had the dialogues memorized?

Perhaps those painful memories would give you the strength to say, "No more!"

Switch off your Imagination

That is probably a horrible thing to tell a person, but necessary in some cases. You see, when you let your imagination go wild, it can literally go wild, thinking up crazy things that mess with your mind. See that couple standing over there talking to each other? They're not just talking; they are criticizing the way you look. See those groups of people laughing at something someone said? Of course they're laughing at you!

So switch off your imagination and live in the reality. When you are at a social gathering, concentrate on you and you only. Talk, mingle, eat, drink, go home! No need to think about what people are thinking about you, or what they will say about you later when you are not there. That's not your problem!

Stop Having Unrealistic Expectations
That's probably one problem almost every human being in this world has - the desire to be perfect and faultless. Not only is that not possible, it's not right to be perfect, but not many of us know this. Some common examples go:
"I need to be perfect so that people will like me!"
"I can't be making mistakes."
"I cannot be anxious; people will find out."
"It is important to be loved by everyone!"

When a person desires to be perfect but cannot achieve their goals, it makes them self-conscious and fearful of the alternative. The most realistic way to avoid social anxiety is to stop having an unrealistic anticipation of life.
Ask the Questions
If you are uncomfortable with sharing your personal information with others, then

stop others from questioning you by asking all the questions yourself. Try to be curious in the other person you are talking to at a social gathering and ask them questions regarding their hobbies, families and careers. This way, you won't have to talk much but just ask the questions, while your acquaintance will do all the talking.

By asking questions and learning about the person, there is a chance that you might also begin to open up to the person more. Knowing personal details about the person might bring them closer to you, and even though you are afraid of meeting new people, you might end up making a new friend.

Adopt a Pet

Pets are amazing for reducing stress and anxiety. They are someone who will accept you for whoever you are and will not need you to be perfect. People can actually be themselves when they are around their pets. Talk to your cat, your dog or your goldfish - practice talking to them as if they are human beings and can understand what you are saying. This will be a great practice until you are confident enough to go and talk to any adult.

Pets can also create enormous opportunities to meet new people, especially when you are taking them out for a run. They are great conversation starters, and many relationships (particularly, romantic ones) have started when two adults with two dogs meet at the doggy park.

Be Yourself

One of the main reasons that social phobia exists is because many people don't like the way they are or the way they think they appear to other people. They think they are dull, uninteresting, boring and not really worth other people taking the time to know better. Most people who experience social anxiety disorder desire to be interesting and attractive to others and when they can't do that, they withdraw more into themselves.

One important tip to give to such people is to 'be themselves'. When they can accept themselves the way they naturally are, they will know to interact with people being themselves and not try to be anyone else.

Start Small

No one is asking you to get on stage at the first try to declare, "To be or not to be, that is the question!" Once you decide to start on the road to delivery, start small. Call up a local bakery and idly question them regarding their opening and closing time; chat up a passenger on the way to work; order a coffee on your own.

Start with a situation, which requires no human contact, such as taking a solitary walk in the park, or watching a movie alone. Afterwards, start with small children and animals - two beings you don't have to be self-conscious with because they will not judge you. Work your way up to adults when you feel confident enough to interact with them.

Stop Negative Thoughts

This tip might sound a little juvenile but it's known to work in many situations. The trick is - whenever you feel any negative thoughts creeping up to your mind, just - STOP! Stop that thought right there, right that moment, and divert your brain somewhere else.

"I'm sure this dress is wrong here; I can feel people -" STOP! "The color combination on the study wall looks amazing! I must remember to compliment the host."

"If I call the waiter again, he would be mad at me. I have already -" STOP! "I've heard the pizza here is awesome. Must try!"

"I shouldn't buy so many chocolates; people are looking at me funny. They must think -" STOP! "I love Twix. Must take a dozen."

The Power of Small Talk

Never underestimate the power of small talk. Sometimes the "Hey, did you see the game last night?" and "Wonderful weather tonight!" can last hours and remove a lot of awkwardness between two people.

When you find yourself alone at a social gathering with a recently introduced stranger and no one to rescue you, small talk can save the day. Start with the weather, the host's generosity, the weather again, the breaking news, the quality of the food and if you begin to feel comfortable, you will find yourself slowly comparing your views on world politics and international cuisine. And voila! This is the beginning of a brand new friendship!

Practice, Practice, Practice

After all, practice makes a man perfect! Practice talking; practice ordering, practice conversing, practice funny stories and jokes, practice famous speeches given hundreds of years ago. Practice while working in front of the mirror with your dog/cat, with a good friend, practice anywhere and everywhere!

If you are planning to ask out someone special, practice your line by yourself or a close friend. Choose your words correctly, to make sure that you don't sound like a zombie when you actually do go and ask. If you are preparing for a presentation for work, gather your family members and practice the speech in front of them.

Many more ideas and tricks will come to you when you start your journey towards freedom from social anxiety disorder.

CHAPTER 25: Beyond the Anxiety Epidemic

Emotional Intelligence
Emotional intelligence is fundamental to survive and flourish and may be more critical than IQ (intelligence quotient) to prevent children from having anxiety and depression, as well as reinforce relationships.

In 1995, the publication of Goleman's best-selling book Emotional Intelligence popularized the idea. Emotional intelligence, also known as emotional leadership, emotional intelligence quotient or emotional quotient (EQ) is the capacity to perceive and comprehend both your emotions and the emotions of others and utilize that data to modify your thinking and behavior.

There are four ways to measure emotional intelligence: the capacity to identify emotions in oneself (intrapersonal) or in others (interpersonal); the capacity to think about the emotion they identify; the capacity to comprehend the emotions; and the capacity to use this information to control their own emotions or behaviors. Actions of a person with high emotional intelligence enhance his/her interpersonal relationships while accomplishing his/her goals.

Emotional intelligence combines at least two of the different types of intelligence, interpersonal and intrapersonal intelligence. Intrapersonal intelligence involves the way you relate to yourself, while interpersonal intelligence invoves the way you relate to others. For example, a young woman who sits in a cubicle and is known as the extremely brainy lady who is too shy to relate to people may be known as the classic nerd. She is logical and mathematically intelligent but not emotionally intelligent. Another girl who is known as the socialite is adored by everyone and the most popular student, but for her, simple algebra may as well be rocket science. She is emotionally intelligent but not logical-mathematically intelligent. Some extroverts are not necessarily emotionally intelligent. For example, a person who is biased, known to trash-talk and harass others, and who everyone hates may express his feelings clearly, but he is not emotionally mature. Persons with high emotional intelligence have an adequate amount of all forms of intelligence. At the other extreme, a person who almost completely lacks emotional intelligence can be considered to have alexithymia.

Emotional (interpersonal and intrapersonal) intelligence is considered to be more essential than academic (logical mathematical) intelligence for greater success in life. It's important to understand why it is more imperative to be emotionally intelligent. Women are generally described as emotional beings. Truthfully, all humans are emotional beings. Successful individuals of all walks of life whether in religious, business, musical or other industries are aware of this. Well-known and successful businessmen Zig Ziglar and Brian Tracy know that people buy based on emotions and justify through logic. This implies we do not think logically but emotionally. We only try to justify our emotions logically. That's why businesses try to be friendly with customers and staff, and musicians try to maintain good relationships with their producers and fans. In many cases, musicians have experienced heavy losses because their fans were not happy with them. In 1966, the band the Beatles suddenly lost popularity in the United States and people were burning their albums because a band member said they were more famous than Jesus, not because people hated their music. They realized the implication of that statement in the United States a little too late at that time. They never really recovered after that public debacle.

Fast forward to now, we frequently hear about stars with millions of fans who have been unfollowed on social media by over one million people at once, not because their music was trashy, but because they did something fans were not satisfied with. Even computer geeks who invent the greatest apps must maintain good relationships with investors and customers. One of the leading causes for a business to fail is poor customer service or inadequate staff motivation which ultimately leads to poor products or customer service.

No matter who someone is, or how successful they are, no one wants people to despise them. People can undeniably do you the most harm when they hate you and can be the most helpful if they love you. A truly successful person is not necessarily the one with a great deal of money but one who, in addition to money, has an upbeat, satisfied life. You cannot really be happy if you don't have good relationships with other people. We are all social creatures.

Teenage girls, whether or not they are college students, not only need emotional intelligence to have a chance at becoming more successful or happy but also need emotional intelligence to become more resilient in conquering mental disorders. Let's be honest; teenage girls face a considerable amount of pressure from parents, school teachers, friends and peers. Maybe it's due to puberty hormones or cultural differences, but millennial girls often feel the people around them don't understand them. This can be discouraging and may prompt nervousness. Possibly, that is why more teenagers are experiencing anxiety, depression and other mental issues and trying to cope with it through harmful practices which may lead to phone addiction, substance abuse, or misconduct.

Some of these coping mechanisms can lower both academic and emotional intelligence. One study has shown that internet addiction lowers emotional intelligence because excessively introverted people become dependent on the internet as a way to avoid social interactions. Indeed, internet addiction lowers emotional intelligence and academic intelligence and has been connected to an increased chance for depression, obsessive compulsive disorders, mood disorders, and a host of other mental issues that can lead to marital, financial, academic and social problems. Studies have also shown that people with high emotional intelligence have a lower propensity to develop mental issues like anxiety and depression. Although for treatment of mental disorders many other factors must be considered, emotional intelligence development may be of great value in treating many mental health issues. The more that parents and teachers pay attention to the emotional intelligence of Gen Z and college students, the more they can help them build resiliency to mental health problems, such as anxiety disorders.

Self-Compassion

Practicing self-compassion is beneficial to your mental wellbeing. Kristin Neff, PhD conducted research on self-compassion and proposed it as a way to reduce anxiety and depression. Low self-esteem, insecure attachments in relationships, and a misguided feeling of loneliness—during which the woman suffering from anxiety thinks she is alone in this world and no one understands how she is suffering—is typically observed in anxiety and depression. Worse still, the woman may even believe that people around her are mocking her and think she is strange which will further isolate her and worsen the anxiety. Self-compassion aims to reduce these thought patterns. Unlike the usual thought patterns present with anxiety, in which the woman negatively criticizes herself and is overdependent on what others think about her, self-compassion directs the anxious woman to love herself.

There are three primary components of self-compassion.

Kindness towards yourself

You may have to stop criticizing yourself. Stop bringing down your self-esteem by being judgmental and recognize you are responsible for your happiness. Being kind to yourself means instead of thinking, "I am a fat pig, and that's why no one wants me," encourage yourself to notice the true beauty inside you and stop hating yourself. It may be helpful to realize that when you love yourself and others, then others will begin to love you. If you don't love yourself, then it may be difficult to love others because you cannot give what you don't have.

Awareness of common humanity

You are not suffering alone and there are other people like you who understand what you are experiencing. This awareness can mean refusing any thought that says you are suffering on your own. It may be helpful to seek a support group of others going through the same problem that you are. You may find that others have possibly been through worse which can help you think better of yourself and of others. Meeting them and learning about their struggles may show you that there are people who understand what you are going through and who care.

Practicing mindfulness

Become aware of the negative thoughts going through your mind and look for positive ways to manage them. This is the most extensively studied part of self-compassion, and it is one of the principles used in cognitive behavior therapy. To deal with a problem, you must be able to identify the problem. Being mindful is becoming aware of those negative and harmful thoughts so you can retrain your mind to think positively instead of being critical. Mindfulness can involve replacing negative thoughts, such as "Oh my gosh, I'm having a relapse," or "I'm never going to get rid of this anxiety problem" with positive alternatives, such as "A relapse can happen to anyone. I'm still on the path of recovery," or "I am getting better day by day."

Studies conducted by Dr. Neff and others have shown that in addition to self-compassion, traits such as self-kindness, common humanity, and mindfulness have also been linked to improved wellbeing. An association was found between self-compassion and a stable sense of self-worth. Self-worth is different from egocentrism or high self-esteem in that it does not depend on achievements or qualities. This is because practicing self-compassion teaches you to accept your shortcomings and anxious thoughts and to know that your value is not determined by your success or failure. While a stable sense of self-esteem is good, egocentrism is unsafe. Some research shows that self-esteem, self-compassion, and self-efficacy are related to each other and are connected to improved wellbeing among Gen Z and Millennials. However, of the three, self-compassion is the most stable predictor of wellbeing.

Nevertheless, studies suggest self-esteem, self-compassion, and self-efficacy can prevent anxiety and depression. Some research also confirms that mindfulness is perhaps the most powerful of the three components of self-compassion and is also the most studied. If practiced correctly, it can effectively reduce personal false beliefs of inadequacy. It can also regulate the negative effects of stress. Studies have also correlated healthy social relationships to wellbeing. Self-compassion not only benefits you, but also others around you as people who are self-compassionate tend to have compassion towards others despite their weaknesses. Just as with love, you cannot give what you do not have. If you are not compassionate towards yourself, you will not be genuinely compassionate toward others. Showing compassion to others despite their shortcomings has been demonstrated to improve social relationships which also enhances mental wellbeing.

Fundamentally, self-compassion can be an excellent way to confront anxiety because it improves some areas in which people with anxiety may be lacking. Results may include boosting self-esteem, reducing false criticisms of oneself and enriching relationships with others.

RESOURCES

National Suicide Prevention Lifeline 1-800-273-TALK (8255)

Anxiety and Depression Association of America https://adaa.org

National Alliance on Mental Illness https://www.nami.org

National Institute of Mental Health https://www.nimh.nih.gov
Centers for Disease Prevention Mental Health https://www.cdc.gov/mentalhealth
American Psychological Association https://www.apa.org

REFERENCES

Acharya, J. P., Acharya, I., & Waghrey, D. (2013). A study on some of the common health effects of cell-phones amongst college students. Journal of Community Medicine & Health Education, 3(214), doi:10.4172/2161-0711.1000214

American Psychiatric Association. (2000). Diagnostic and statistical manual of mental disorders (4th ed., text rev.). Washington, DC: Author.

American Psychological Association. (2015). APA review confirms link between playing violent video games and aggression.

American Psychiatric Association. (2013). Diagnostic and statistical manual of mental disorders (5th ed.). (p. 189). Arlington, VA: American Psychiatric Publishing.

Anxiety and Depression Association of America. Facts & Statistics. Retrieved from https://adaa.org/about-adaa/press-room/facts-statistics

Beck, J. S. (2011). Cognitive behavior therapy basics and beyond. New York: The Guilford Press.

Boumosleh, J. M., & Jaalouk, D. (2017). Depression, anxiety, and smartphone addiction in university students- A cross-sectional study. PLOS ONE, doi:10.1371/journal.pone.0182239

Budinger, M. C., Drazdowski, T. K., & Ginsburg, G. S. (2013). Anxiety-promoting parenting behaviors: a comparison of anxious parents with and without social anxiety disorder. Child Psychiatry and Human Development, 44(3), 412–418. doi:10.1007/s10578-012-0335-9

Burstein, M., & Ginsburg, G. S. (2010). The effect of parental modeling of anxious behaviors and cognitions in school-aged children: An experimental pilot study. Behaviour Research and Therapy, 48(6), 506–515. doi:10.1016/j.brat.2010.02.006

Gardner, H. (1983). Frames of mind: The theory of multiple intelligences. NYC: Basic Books.

Goleman, D. (2005). Emotional intelligence: Why it can matter more than IQ. New York: Bantam Books.

Gruttadaro, D., Crudo, D. (2012). College students speak: A survey report on mental health. NAMI, the National Alliance on Mental Illness. https://www.nami.org/About-NAMI/Publications-Reports/Survey-Reports

Harvard Health Publishing. (2015, October). Two types of drugs you may want to avoid for the sake of your brain. Retrieved from https://www.health.harvard.edu/mind-and-mood/two-types-of-drugs-you-may-want-to-avoid-for-the-sake-of-your-brain

Heath, C., & Heath, D. (2010). Switch: How to change things when change is hard. United States: Broadway Books.

Hertz, N. (2016). Think millennials have it tough? For 'Generation K', life is even harsher. Retrieved from https://www.theguardian.com/world/2016/mar/19/think-millennials-have-it-tough-for-generation-k-life-is-even-harsher

Mattheisen, M., Samuels, J. F., Wang, Y., Greenberg, B. D., Fyer, A. J., McCracken, J. T. et al. Genome-wide association study in obsessive-compulsive disorder: results from the OCGAS. Molecular Psychiatry, 20(3), 337-344, doi:10.1038/mp.2014.43

McLean, C. P., Asnaani, A., Litz, B. T., & Hofmann, S. G. (2012) Gender differences in anxiety disorders: prevalence, course of illness, comorbidity and burden of illness. Journal of Psychiatric Research, 45(8), 1027–1035.

Na, H. R., Kang, E. H., Lee, J. H., & Yu, B. H. (2011). The genetic basis of panic disorder.

Journal of Korean Medical Science, 26(6), 701-710. doi:10.3346/jkms.2011.26.6.701

Neff, K. (2011). Self-compassion: The proven power of being kind to yourself. New York, NY: HarperCollins.

Raes, F., Pommier, E., Neff, K. D., & Van Gucht, D. (2011). Construction and factorial validation of a short form of the self-compassion scale. Clinical Psychology & Psychotherapy. 18, 250-255.

Remes, O., Brayne, C., van der Linde, R., & Lafortune, L. (2016). A systematic review of reviews on the prevalence of anxiety disorders in adult populations. Brain and Behavior, 6(7), e00497. doi:10.1002/brb3.497

Twenge, J. M. (2017). iGen: Why today's super-connected kids are growing up less rebellious, more tolerant, less happy—and completely unprepared for adulthood—and what that means for the rest of us. Atria Books.

Walsh, R. (2011, October). Lifestyle and mental health. American Psychologist, 66(7), 579-592.

Wilber, K., Patten, T., Leonard, D., & Morelli, M. (2008). Integral life practice: A 21st-century blueprint for physical health, emotional balance, mental clarity, and spiritual awakening. Integral Books.

World Health Organization. (2009). Pharmacological treatment of mental disorders in primary health care. Retrieved November 20, 2016, from https://www.ncbi.nlm.nih.gov/books/NBK 143202/pdf/Bookshelf_NBK143202.pdf

Chapter 26: Obsessive-Compulsive Disorder: When Unwanted Thoughts or Irresistible Actions Take Over

Do you constantly have disturbing uncontrollable thoughts? Do you feel the urge to repeat the same behaviors or rituals over and over? Are these thoughts and behaviors making it hard for you to do things you enjoy?

If so, you may have obsessive-compulsive disorder (OCD). The good news is that, with treatment, you can overcome the fears and behaviors that may be putting your life on hold.

What is it like to have OCD?

"I couldn't do anything without my rituals. They invaded every aspect of my life. Counting really bogged me down. I would wash my hair three times because three was a good luck number for me. It took me longer to read because I'd have to count the lines in a paragraph. When I set my alarm at night, I had to set it to a time that wouldn't add up to a 'bad' number."

"Getting dressed in the morning was tough because I had to follow my routine or I would become very anxious and start getting dressed all over again." I always worried that if I didn't follow my routine, my parents were going to die. These thoughts triggered more anxiety and more rituals. Because of the time I spent on rituals, I was unable to do a lot of things that were important to me. I couldn't seem to overcome them until I got treatment."

What is OCD?

OCD is a common, chronic (long-lasting) disorder in which a person has uncontrollable, reoccurring thoughts (obsessions) and behaviors (compulsions) that he or she feels the urge to repeat over and over in response to the obsession.

While everyone sometimes feels the need to double check things, people with OCD have uncontrollable thoughts that cause them anxiety, urging them to check things repeatedly or perform routines and rituals for at least 1 hour per day. Performing the routines or rituals may bring brief but temporary relief from the anxiety. However, left untreated, these thoughts and rituals cause the person great distress and get in the way of work, school, and personal relationships.

What are the signs and symptoms of OCD?

People with OCD may have obsessions, compulsions, or both. Some people with OCD also have a tic disorder. Motor tics are sudden, brief, repetitive movements, such as eye blinking, facial grimacing, shoulder shrugging, or head or shoulder jerking. Common vocal tics include repetitive throat-clearing, sniffing, or grunting sounds.

Obsessions may include:

- Fear of germs or contamination
- Fear of losing or misplacing something

- Worries about harm coming towards oneself or others
- Unwanted and taboo thoughts involving sex, religion, or others
- Having things symmetrical or in perfect order

Compulsions may include:

- Excessively cleaning or washing a body part
- Keeping or hoarding unnecessary objects
- Ordering or arranging items in a particular, precise way
- Repeatedly checking on things, such as making sure that the door is locked or the oven is off
- Repeatedly counting items
- Constantly seeking reassurance

What causes OCD?

OCD may have a genetic component. It sometimes runs in families, but no one knows for sure why some family members have it while others don't. OCD usually begins in adolescence or young adulthood, and tends to appear at a younger age in boys than in girls. Researchers have found that several parts of the brain, as well as biological processes, play a key role in obsessive thoughts and compulsive behavior, as well as the fear and anxiety related to them. Researchers also know that people who have suffered physical or sexual trauma are at an increased risk for OCD.

Some children may develop a sudden onset or worsening of OCD symptoms after a streptococcal infection; this post-infectious autoimmune syndrome is called Pediatric Autoimmune Neuropsychiatric Disorder Associated with Streptococcal Infections (PANDAS).

How is OCD treated?

The first step is to talk with your doctor or health care provider about your symptoms. The clinician should do an exam and ask you about your health history to make sure that a physical problem is not causing your symptoms. Your doctor may refer you to a mental health specialist, such as a psychiatrist, psychologist, social worker, or counselor for further evaluation or treatment.

OCD is generally treated with cognitive behavior therapy, medication, or both. Speak with your mental health professional about the best treatment for you.

Cognitive behavioral therapy (CBT)

In general, CBT teaches you different ways of thinking, behaving, and reacting to the obsessions and compulsions.

Exposure and Response Prevention (EX/RP) is a specific form of CBT which has been shown to help many patients recover from OCD. EX/RP involves gradually exposing you to your fears or obsessions and teaching you healthy ways to deal with the anxiety they cause.

Other therapies, such as habit reversal training, can also help you overcome compulsions.

For children, mental health professionals can also identify strategies to manage stress and increase support to avoid exacerbating OCD symptoms in school and home settings.

Medication
Doctors also may prescribe different types of medications to help treat OCD including selective serotonin reuptake inhibitors (SSRIs) and a type of serotonin reuptake inhibitor (SRI) called clomipramine.

SSRIs and SRIs are commonly used to treat depression, but they are also helpful for the symptoms of OCD. SSRIs and SRIs may take 10 – 12 weeks to start working, longer than is required for the treatment of depression. These medications may also cause side effects, such as headaches, nausea, or difficulty sleeping.

People taking clomipramine, which is in a different class of medication from the SSRIs, sometimes experience dry mouth, constipation, rapid heartbeat, and dizziness on standing. These side effects are usually not severe for most people and improve as treatment continues, especially if the dose starts off low and is increased slowly over time. Talk to your doctor about any side effects that you have. Don't stop taking your medication without talking to your doctor first. Your doctor will work with you to find the best medication and dose for you.

Don't give up on treatment too quickly. Both psychotherapy and medication can take some time to work. While there is no cure for OCD, current treatments enable most people with this disorder to control their symptoms and lead full, productive lives. A healthy lifestyle that involves relaxation and managing stress can also help combat OCD. Make sure to also get enough sleep and exercise, eat a healthy diet, and turn to family and friends whom you trust for support.

Chapter 27: SOUND MEDITATION

Okay, white bread me is going to go Asian on you again by introducing you to meditation. But instead of sitting with our eyes closed trying not to think of anything, we will be using what's called a mantra, a word or phrase that is repeated over and over. The Universe is energy. So is sound. Repeating certain words or phrases over and over in your mind or out loud joins us with that universal energy and counteracts thoughts that produce anxiety.

If you're like me and your brain refuses to shut up when your trying to relax for sleep, this might be the answer for you. You can chose any word, but it's best to use positive words such as peace, love, joy or whatever one word you find pleasant.

The beauty of using a mantra is it has no side-effects like sleep medications. Deep breathing, mantras, yoga, tai chi all can be used to quiet a restless mind and relax tension. And when you wake up in the middle of the night, you can use them to get back to sleep faster - always a bonus.

A series of slow, flowing body movements, tai chi emphasizes concentration, relaxation and the conscious circulation of vital energy throughout the body. If you've ever hung out in a park and noticed a group of people slowly moving in synch, you've probably witnessed tai chi. And why are you hanging out in a park? Started from martial arts, today it is a way of calming the mind, conditioning the body, and reducing stress., with focus on their breathing and keeping their attention in the present moment.

Safe for all ages and fitness levels including seniors, kids and anyone recovering from injuries, Tai chi is a like yoga, once you've learned the basics you can practice alone or with others. The benefits of learning these relaxation techniques is ginormous.

Do them as part of your relaxation routine or if you wake up in the middle of the night.

(back to top)
REDUCE MENTAL STRESS

- Use a journal to record worries and concerns before you retire

- Check off tasks on your to-do list that you finished, jot down what you want to do tomorrow and then forget it - let go!

- Calming music - not rock-n-roll (unfortunately), rap, heavy metal or punk - I'm sure you get it why.

- Read a 'real' book that makes you feel relaxed - not an ebook

- Talk with a friend or therapist about what's bugging you.

Don't stress
Make relaxation your goal
Do a quiet, non-stimulating activity
Postpone worrying

Conclusion

In this handbook we've tried to show you just some of the many, many ways that anxiety can be treated. If you take nothing else away from this, please just know that you are not alone.

There are millions in the world feeling just as "alone" as you do. There is help out there and it comes in many forms. Surround yourself with those you love and who you care about. Those who care about you, in return, will be there throughout this tough-but-manageable ordeal.

Just as they require patience to help you with your anxiety, you must take the time to try and educate them, as well as yourself, about all that your anxiety can encompass.

It can be a short road and it can be a long road but it never, ever...ever...has to be a road you travel alone.

Please educate yourself and see a doctor as soon as possible. Many of the techniques and methods mentioned in this handbook can be done at home but should be done with a doctor's supervision to ensure no adverse reactions result. Again, there may be underlying medical conditions causing your anxiety. Call your doctor today!

Good luck!!

Lightning Source UK Ltd.
Milton Keynes UK
UKHW020801191222
414157UK00015B/1036